HEALTH SCIENCES IMPLEMENTATION BLUEPRINT (HSIB)

A Clinical Guide to Translating Evidence into Practice

for Advanced Medical Students and Early-Career Residents

DR. G.L. KESLING

HEALTH SCIENCES IMPLEMENTATION BLUEPRINT

ISBN: 979-8-234-05925-3
May 2026

DEDICATION

"To him who devotes his life to science, nothing can give more happiness than increasing the number of discoveries; but his cup of joy is full when the results of his studies immediately find practical applications."

— Louis Pasteur, 1882

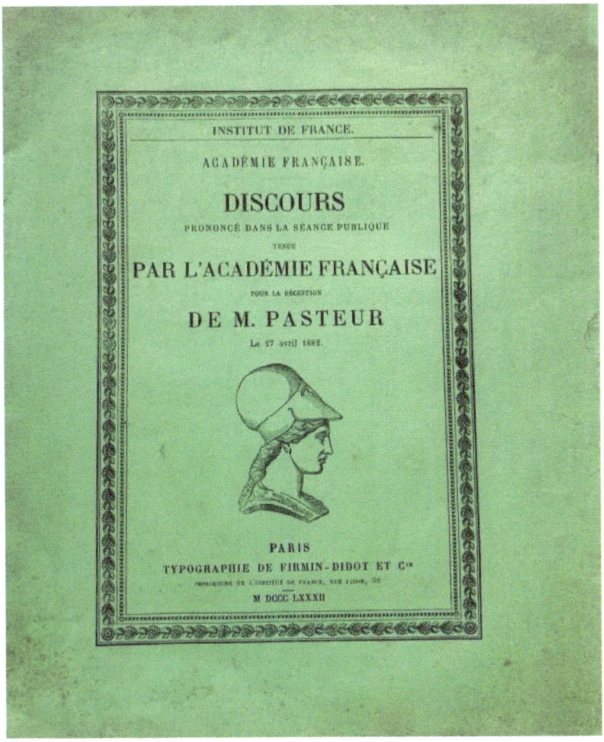

FIGURE *Pasteur's 1882 Discours de réception à l'Académie française.*

In his 1882 Discours de réception à l'Académie française, Pasteur wrote that the scientist "cares little for glory" and is filled with joy when his discoveries yield "fruits useful to humanity." Earlier, in his 1854 inaugural lecture at Douai, he emphasized that there are no "applied sciences," only "applications of science," underscoring the inseparability of inquiry and practical benefit.

PREFACE

The Implementation Gap You're Already Seeing

The evidence-based guideline that nobody follows. The discharge protocol exists on paper but not in practice. The screening tool that should be used but is not. The innovation that worked at the academic center is down the road, but it does not seem to be gaining traction at your institution. The patient who did not get the care they needed—not because we do not know what works, but because the system failed to deliver it.

This is the implementation gap, and it is costly. Despite decades of rigorous research producing evidence-based interventions, the systematic uptake of these practices into routine clinical care continues to lag, often taking 17 years or more to translate research findings into widespread practice. [1] For patients with conditions like heart failure, fewer than half receive guideline-directed medical therapy, and disparities in implementation are even more pronounced among historically marginalized populations. [2-3]

As a senior medical student or early-career resident, you are uniquely positioned to address this gap. You have fresh eyes on broken systems, protected time for improvement projects, direct patient contact that reveals implementation barriers, and the credibility to question "the way we've always done it." Implementation science—the study of methods for increasing the systematic uptake of evidence-based interventions in clinical practice—gives you the tools to turn your observations into action. [2-3]

This handbook introduces you to the Health Sciences Implementation Blueprint (HSIB), a practical framework designed for clinicians who want to close the gap between evidence and practice. Whether you're designing a required QI project, leading a resident-driven initiative, or trying to improve care for your patients, this guide will help you translate research into reality.

TABLE OF CONTENTS

Health Sciences Implementation Blueprint

CHAPTER 8

CHAPTER 9

APPENDIX

CHAPTER INTRODUCTION

Implementation Science for Clinicians

What Is Implementation Science?

Implementation science is the study of methods to promote the systematic uptake of research findings and other evidence-based practices into routine practice, thereby improving the quality and effectiveness of health services. [2-3] It answers the question every clinician asks: "We know what works, why isn't it happening, and how do we fix it?"

This differs from traditional clinical research in critical ways:

TABLE 1 Traditional clinical research and implementation science compared

TRADITIONAL CLINICAL RESEARCH	IMPLEMENTATION SCIENCE
Does this intervention work?	How do we get this intervention to work in the real world?
Efficacy under ideal conditions	Effectiveness in routine practice
Highly controlled protocols	Pragmatic, adaptable designs
Homogeneous populations	Diverse, real-world populations
Primary outcome: clinical effectiveness	Primary outcomes: adoption, fidelity, sustainability

Implementation studies often use pragmatic designs that allow flexibility in protocols to tailor interventions in real time as they are being used, increasing external validity and the likelihood that interventions will be adopted, implemented correctly, and maintained. [3]

Why This Matters to You Now

You are already doing implementation work—you just may not call it that. Every time you:

- Wonder why the sepsis package is not being completed consistently.
- Try to improve handoffs between your team and the night float.
- Advocate for a patient who cannot afford their medications.
- Notice that discharge summaries are not reaching primary care physicians.
- Question why evidence-based depression screening is not happening in your clinic.

...you are identifying implementation problems.

The difference between frustration and impact lies in the use of a systematic approach to addressing them. Here is why the implementation of science skills is essential for your career:

Residency programs require QI participation

Most residency programs in the U.S., Canada, and the U.K. require residents to complete quality improvement projects as part of training and advancement. [6] The ACGME requires all residents to demonstrate competency in practice-based learning and improvement and systems-based practice.

You can improve patient outcomes now

Resident-led QI initiatives have demonstrated significant improvements in clinical outcomes, including reduced catheter-associated bloodstream infections, improved medication reconciliation, decreased door-to-balloon times for STEMI, and enhanced transitions of care.

You will be a systems leader

Whether you pursue **academic medicine, community practice, or hospital leadership**, your role will extend far beyond individual patient care. You will be expected to **lead improvement efforts that strengthen systems**, **serve on interdisciplinary committees that shape institutional priorities**, **implement new clinical and operational protocols**, and **contribute to the ongoing cycle of organizational learning and innovation**.

In academic medicine, this means translating evidence into practice—designing and evaluating educational programs, mentoring colleagues, and aligning departmental goals with broader institutional missions. In community practice, it involves identifying population-level needs, coordinating care across diverse settings, and fostering partnerships that advance equity and access. In hospital leadership, it requires integrating data-driven decision-making with frontline insight, ensuring that quality improvement initiatives are sustainable, measurable, and responsive to patient outcomes.

Across all these domains, clinicians are called to act as **agents of change**—to bridge the gap between knowledge and performance, to cultivate cultures of safety and collaboration, and to model continuous professional development. Leadership in medicine today demands fluency in improvement science, systems thinking, and ethical stewardship. It is not merely about managing processes but about **mobilizing people and ideas** toward shared goals that enhance care, learning, and community well-being.

Ultimately, your capacity to lead these efforts defines your contribution to the profession itself: transforming data into knowledge, knowledge into performance, and performance into better health for the populations you serve.
[1][7]

Health parity demands of implementation science

Biopsychosocial disparities in cardiovascular disease, maternal mortality, diabetes, and every other condition are not primarily due to lack of knowledge about what works—they are due to failures of implementation in under-resourced settings and for marginalized populations. [3] Implementation science provides the tools to address structural barriers and achieve equity.

An international, multidisciplinary study of eighty-two implementation experts conducted across multiple countries and health systems identified the most essential competencies for conducting both implementation practice and implementation research. [4] This work is foundational because it clarifies the distinct yet overlapping skill sets clinicians and scholars need to move evidence into routine care and to study the processes that make such movement successful.

For **implementation practice**—the day-to-day work clinicians perform when integrating new evidence-based interventions into real clinical environments—experts emphasized three core domains: **collaboration**, **knowledge**, and **skills**. Collaboration refers not only to working effectively with colleagues but also to engaging patients, families, administrators, and community partners as co-producers of change. Knowledge encompasses understanding the evidence base, the local context, and the mechanisms through which interventions exert their effects. Skills include the practical abilities required to adapt interventions, troubleshoot barriers, communication across disciplines, and sustain improvement over time. These competencies reflect the reality that clinicians are central actors in implementation: they must navigate complex systems, negotiate competing priorities, and translate abstract recommendations into workable, context-sensitive practices.

For **implementation research**, experts identified a slightly different constellation of priorities: **research methodology**, **knowledge**, and **skills**. Research methodology includes rigorous study design, measurement, analytic strategies, and the ability to evaluate implementation outcomes such as fidelity, adoption, reach, and sustainability. Knowledge refers to mastery of implementation theories, frameworks, and models that guide hypothesis generation and interpretation. Skills encompass the capacity to conduct mixed-methods research, engage stakeholders in co-design, manage data, and disseminate findings in ways that influence policy and practice. Together, these competencies position implementation researchers to generate generalizable insights about how best to integrate evidence into diverse settings and populations. [4]

To support the development of these competencies, a comprehensive framework for training health professionals in implementation and dissemination science proposes **seven interrelated domains** that together form a developmental roadmap for learners at all levels. [5] These domains reflect the interdisciplinary, context-dependent, and relational nature of implementation work:

1. **Team Science** – This domain emphasizes the ability to lead and collaborate across disciplines, professions, and organizational hierarchies. Effective implementation requires shared mental models, psychological safety, and the capacity to integrate diverse expertise—from clinicians and researchers to administrators, community partners, and patients. Team science prepares learners to navigate these dynamics and to cultivate high-functioning, cross-sector partnerships.
2. **Context Identification** – Implementation success depends heavily on understanding the specific environment in which change will occur. This includes organizational culture, leadership support, workflow patterns, resource availability, and structural barriers. Learners develop the ability to conduct contextual assessments, identify leverage points, and tailor interventions to local realities without compromising core components.
3. **Literature Identification and Assessment** – Because implementation is evidence-driven, learners must be able to rapidly locate, appraise, and synthesize research findings. This domain includes skills in systematic searching, critical appraisal, and translating evidence into actionable guidance. It also prepares learners to identify gaps in literature that may require adaptation or innovation.

4. **Community Engagement** – Implementation efforts are most effective when they are co-designed with the people they aim to serve. This domain focuses on partnering with patients, families, community organizations, and other stakeholders to ensure cultural relevance, acceptability, and sustainability. It emphasizes shared decision-making, bidirectional communication, and respect for lived experience.
5. **Intervention Design and Research Implementation** – Learners develop the ability to adapt evidence-based practices to local contexts while maintaining fidelity to the mechanisms that make them effective. This includes planning, piloting, refining, and scaling interventions; coordinating logistics; and integrating implementation strategies such as training, audit-and-feedback, or workflow redesign.
6. **Evaluation of the Effect of Translational Activity** – This domain focuses on measuring what matters. Learners gain expertise in selecting and applying implementation outcomes (e.g., adoption, fidelity, penetration, sustainability), designing evaluation plans, and using data to guide iterative improvement. This competency ensures that implementation efforts are not only enacted but also assessed for impact and equity.
7. **Behavioral Change Communication Strategies** – Because implementation ultimately requires people to change what they do, learners must understand how to promote adoption and sustainment through effective communication. This includes framing messages, tailoring communication to different audiences, using feedback loops, and applying behavioral science principles to support long-term change.

Together, these seven domains provide a comprehensive structure for preparing clinicians, researchers, and leaders to advance implementation and dissemination science. They highlight that successful implementation is not merely a technical task but a relational, contextual, and iterative process that requires a blend of scientific rigor, practical skill, and collaborative leadership.

Implementation Science Competencies for Residents

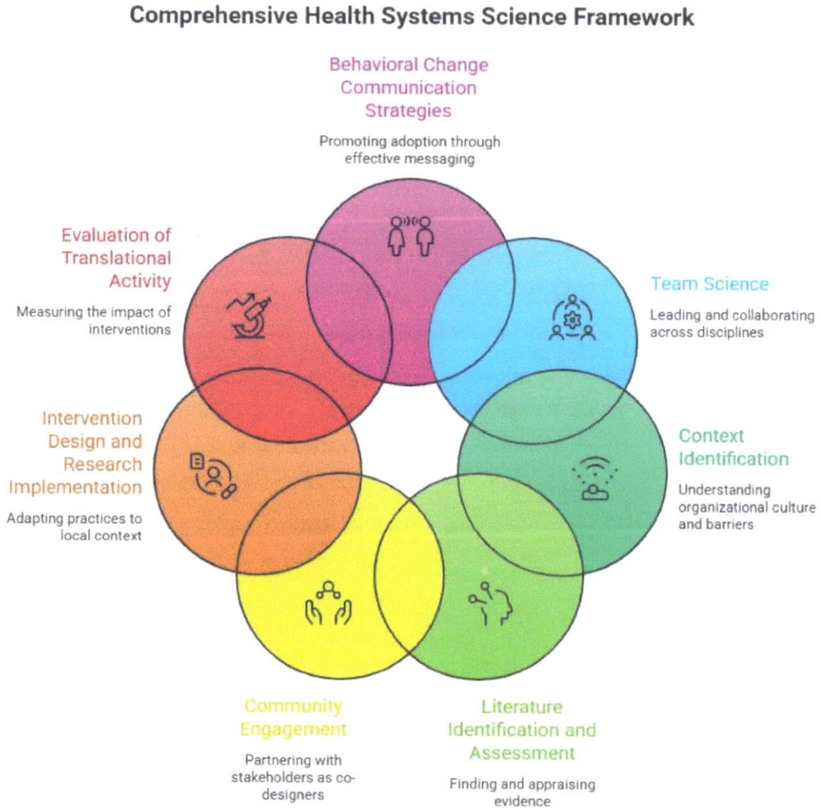

FIGURE *1 The seven competency domains for implementation practice and research.*

These competencies align closely with Health Systems Science (HSS), now recognized as the third pillar of medical education alongside basic and clinical sciences. [8-9] HSS encompasses systems thinking, value-based care, population health, informatics, quality improvement, and interprofessional collaboration.

CHAPTER 1

Core Principles of the HSIB

1.1 Data as a Catalyst for Action

The HSIB represents a fundamental shift in how we think about data in clinical practice. Rather than viewing data as static information to be observed and archived, the HSIB treats data as a catalyst for logical actions that drive systemic improvements through active stewardship.

This perspective recognizes that information itself has no inherent value—it's worth lies in its ability to inform decisions, guide interventions, and drive meaningful change. As a clinician, this means that every clinical observation, patient interaction, and system inefficiency you notice represents potential data that can fuel improvement. The implementation of science skills transforms passive observation into active stewardship.

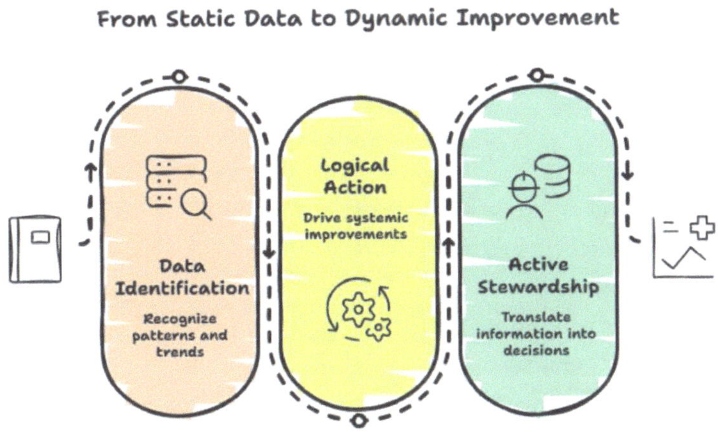

FIGURE *1.1 From static data to dynamic improvement: the active stewardship loop.*

1.2 First-Order Principles: Defining the Problem

Before any meaningful improvement can occur, you must clearly define what you are trying to change. HSIB's first-order principles provide the conceptual foundation for problem definition through four key concepts: facts, properties, relationships, and rules.

Facts

Facts are the verifiable observations about clinical care delivery. These include patient outcomes, process measures, resource utilization, and stakeholder experiences. In your QI work, you might encounter facts such as readmission rates, medication adherence percentages, or patient satisfaction scores. The key is to distinguish between facts (what is actually happening) and assumptions (what we think is happening).

Concepts (Definition of Things) – Precise delineation of entities to ensure clarity.

Clinical example: When implementing a heart failure discharge bundle, you must clearly define:

- What constitutes "heart failure with reduced ejection fraction?"
- What is "guideline-directed medical therapy" (which four medication classes)?
- What defines "successful discharge" (medication reconciliation, follow-up scheduled, patient education completed)?

Properties

Properties are the characteristics that define and describe clinical phenomena. When you encounter a clinical problem, ask yourself: what are its defining properties? For example, when addressing hospital-acquired infections, properties might include infection type, patient population, time of onset, severity, and associated risk factors.

Properties (Attributes of Facts) – Measurable characteristics that inform decision-making. [2-3]

Clinical example: For a sepsis protocol, relevant properties include:

- Time to antibiotic administration (efficacy)
- Percentage of eligible patients who receive the bundle (reach)
- Cost per patient (resource use)
- Nurse satisfaction with the protocol (acceptability)
- Differences in implementation by patient race/ethnicity (equity)

Relationships

Relationships describe how different facts and properties interact with each other. In healthcare, almost nothing happens in isolation—medications interact with comorbidities, social determinants affect treatment adherence, and provider workflows influence patient outcomes. Mapping these relationships reveals leverage points for intervention.

Relationships (Nodes and Edges) – Interconnections between elements that form networks for knowledge flow and collaboration.

Clinical example: For improving stroke care, map the relationships:

- EMS → ED triage → CT scan → neurology consult → interventional radiology
- Identify where delays occur (weak edges) and who controls each step (key nodes)

Rules

Rules are the principles, protocols, and guidelines that govern clinical practice. These include evidence-based recommendations, institutional policies, regulatory requirements, and professional standards. Understanding which rules apply—and where they conflict or fall short—is essential for effective improvement.

Rules (Constraints from Micro to Macro) – Guidelines that scale from individual behaviors to population-level policies.
Clinical example: For opioid prescribing:

- Micro: Individual prescriber habits and patient expectations
- Meso: Departmental protocols and EHR hard stops
- Macro: State prescription drug monitoring programs and CDC guidelines

1.3 Second-Order Principles: Reasoning and Integration

Once you have established the first-order foundation, second-order principles guide how you reason about the problem and integrate evidence to design solutions. These include knowledge representations, reasoning patterns, and information integration strategies.

> ### *KEY INSIGHT*
>
> The HSIB treats data not as a record of what has happened, but as a trigger for what should happen next. The clinician who notices that the sepsis bundle is completed in only 60% of eligible cases is in possession of a fact that demands action; properties (which bundle elements are missed most often), relationships (which units fall short), and rules (institutional protocols and Surviving Sepsis guidelines) together specify the shape of that action.

Building on first-order elements, **second-order principles** enable you to synthesize information and make inferences: [1]
Knowledge Representations – Structured depictions of data, such as frameworks, taxonomies, or models.

Clinical example: Using the Consolidated Framework for Implementation Research (CFIR) to organize barriers to implementing a new clinical pathway across five domains: intervention characteristics, outer setting, inner setting, characteristics of individuals, and process.
Reasoning (Inference & Integration) – Logical processes for drawing conclusions and combining disparate data sources.

Clinical example: Integrating EHR data showing low rates of diabetes screening with qualitative interviews revealing that residents do not know how to order HbA1c tests in the outpatient setting, leading to the inference that the problem is not knowledge but workflow design.

Spatial Models – Methods to compare systems, organize classifications, and group populations:

- **Equivalence**: Comparing outcomes across sites to identify best practices
- **Hierarchical**: Organizing interventions by prevention level (primary, secondary, tertiary)
- **Associative**: Grouping high-risk cohorts for targeted interventions (e.g., patients with HFrEF not on beta-blockers)

CHAPTER 2

Essential Implementation Frameworks

2.1 RE-AIM: The Most Practical Framework for Clinicians

RE-AIM stands for Reach, Effectiveness, Adoption, Implementation, and Maintenance. It is one of the most widely used frameworks for planning and evaluating implementation efforts because it forces you to think beyond "did it work?" to "who did it reach, was it adopted, was it implemented correctly, and was it sustained?"

Reach

The proportion of the target population that participates in the intervention. Ask: Who is receiving this intervention? Who is missing? Example: If you implement a diabetes self-management program, reach is the percentage of eligible patients who actually enroll. A common finding is 45% enrollment but with a significant disparity by ethnicity (32% Hispanic vs 58% non-Hispanic White, $p < 0.01$), suggesting that the recruitment process is not equitable.

Effectiveness

The impact of the intervention on outcomes in a real-world setting (as distinguished from efficacy under controlled trial conditions). Ask: Does it work when delivered by busy clinicians in routine practice? This is the principal source of disappointment in many implementation efforts, in which an intervention shown to work in a randomised trial fails to reproduce its effects in operational settings.

Adoption

The proportion of settings, providers, or organizations that take up the intervention. Ask: Which sites and which clinicians have adopted the intervention? This frequently reveals that adoption is concentrated among the better-resourced sites and more enthusiastic early adopters, and that the population most in need of intervention is least likely to have access to it.

Implementation

How the intervention is actually delivered, including fidelity to design and any adaptations introduced. The relevant questions are whether the protocol was followed as designed and what costs in time and resources were incurred.

Maintenance

The degree to which the intervention is sustained after external support has ended. Ask: Six months after the research team has departed, is the program still in operation? This is the test of whether an improvement has become a permanent feature of the system or has dissipated into the routine.

RE-AIM stands for:

R – Reach

- **Question:** Who participated, and who did not?
- **Clinical application:** If you implement a diabetes self-management program, what percentage of eligible patients enrolled? Were there disparities by race, language, insurance status, or health literacy?
- **Metric example:** 45% of eligible patients with HbA1c >9% enrolled; Hispanic patients were significantly less likely to enroll (32% vs. 58%, $p<0.01$)

E – Effectiveness

- **Question:** What is the impact on outcomes in the real-world setting?
- **Clinical application:** Did the intervention work when delivered by busy residents in a safety-net clinic, not just in a controlled trial?
- **Metric example:** Among enrolled patients, mean HbA1c decreased from 9.8% to 8.2% over 6 months.

A – Adoption

- **Question:** Which settings and staff adopted the intervention?
- **Clinical application:** Did all clinic sites implement the program, or only the most resourced ones? Did all providers participate, or only the enthusiastic early adopters?
- **Metric example:** 3 of 5 clinic sites adopted the program; sites with embedded pharmacists were more likely to adopt.

I – Implementation

- **Question:** How was the intervention delivered? What adaptations occurred?
- **Clinical application:** Was the protocol followed as designed (fidelity), or did teams modify it? What were the costs in time and resources?
- **Metric example:** Only 60% of sessions included all planned components; residents cited time constraints; average cost per patient was $180.

M – Maintenance

- **Question:** Was the intervention sustained after external support ended?
- **Clinical application:** Six months after the research team left, is the program still running? Are outcomes maintained?
- **Metric example:** At 12 months post-implementation, only 1 of 3 sites continued the program; that site had secured ongoing funding for a health educator.

Why RE-AIM matters: It forces you to think beyond "Did it work?" to "Did it reach the right people? Can we sustain it? What did it really cost?" These are the questions that determine whether your QI project becomes standard practice or fades away.

2.2 Implementation Outcomes: What to Measure

Beyond clinical outcomes (patient health improvements), implementation science measures distinct outcomes that tell you whether your intervention is being used as intended. The Proctor framework identifies eight key implementation outcomes:

- **Acceptability** – Do stakeholders find it agreeable?
- **Adoption** – Are providers and patients using it?
- **Appropriateness** – Does it fit the context?
- **Feasibility** – Can it be delivered with available resources?
- **Fidelity** – Is it delivered as intended?
- **Penetration** – Is it integrated into routine practice?
- **Sustainability** – Will it continue after the implementation period?
- **Cost** – What resources does it require?

Implementation Outcome	Definition	Resident-Friendly Measurement	Clinical Example
Acceptability	Stakeholder support for the intervention	Survey: "This protocol is acceptable to me" (1-5 scale)	Nurses rate new sepsis bundles 4.2/5
Adoption	Proportion using the intervention	% of eligible providers/sites that adopt	12 of 15 attendings use the new order set (80%)
Appropriateness	Fit to the setting and population	Survey: "This intervention fits our workflow."	Residents rate telehealth protocol 2.8/5 (poor fit)

Implementation Outcome	Definition	Resident-Friendly Measurement	Clinical Example
Feasibility	Extent intervention can be delivered as intended	% of attempts that succeed	Discharge checklist completed for 65% of patients
Fidelity	Adherence to protocol as designed	% of protocol components completed	Only 3 of 5 bundle elements completed consistently
Penetration	Integration into routine practice	% of eligible patients who receive intervention	Forty percent of eligible diabetics receive a foot exam
Sustainability	Maintenance over time	Outcome measured 6-12 months post-implementation	Hand hygiene compliance sustained at 85% in 1 year
Cost	Resources required	Time, money, personnel	15 minutes per patient; $200 in supplies per month

Practical tip: For your QI project, choose 2-3 implementation outcomes to track alongside your clinical outcome. For example, if you are implementing a delirium screening protocol, measure:

- **Clinical outcome:** % of ICU patients who develop delirium.
- **Adoption:** % of nurses who use the CAM-ICU tool
- **Fidelity:** % of shifts where screening is completed as intended
- **Sustainability:** Are nurses still using it 6 months later

2.3 The Spectrum of Outcomes Framework

Implementation efforts can be classified along three dimensions: temporal phase (immediate, transitional, tertiary), measurement scale (clinical, patient-reported, resource, parity), and prevention scope (primary, secondary, tertiary).

The **Spectrum of Outcomes Framework** [1]helps you think about interventions across time and prevention levels: [1][11]
Sequencing (Timing and Transitions) – Aligning interventions with critical windows:

- **Immediate:** Acute response (e.g., ED management of acute MI)
- **Transitional:** Intermediate care (e.g., hospital-to-home transitions, medication reconciliation, early follow-up)
- **Tertiary:** Long-term management (e.g., cardiac rehab, chronic disease monitoring)

Clinical application: When designing a heart failure readmission reduction initiative, you need interventions at all three levels:

- *Immediate:* Optimize inpatient diuresis and initiate GDMT
- *Transitional:* Ensure 7-day follow-up, medication reconciliation, and teach-back of discharge instructions
- *Tertiary:* Enroll in disease management program, address social determinants (food, housing, transportation)

[1] Concept see: Kesling, G.L. *Better is Possible: Rewiring Leadership for a Networking Future, The Orthogonality of Embedded Design* (2025) ISBN 9798264803574

Scale (Multidimensional Measurement) – Measuring what matters to patients, clinicians, and systems:

- Clinical outcomes (mortality, readmissions, HbA1c)
- Patient-reported outcomes (quality of life, symptom burden, satisfaction)
- Resource utilization (length of stay, ED visits, costs)
- Parity metrics (biopsychosocial disparities by race, ethnicity, language, insurance, zip code)

Scope (Prevention Continuum) – Integrating interventions across primary, secondary, and tertiary prevention:

- **Primary prevention:** Vaccination, health promotion, risk factor modification (e.g., smoking cessation, hypertension control)
- **Secondary prevention:** Screening, early detection, lifestyle intervention (e.g., colonoscopy, mammography, prediabetes management)
- **Tertiary prevention:** Comprehensive disease management, disability limitation (e.g., heart failure clinics, stroke rehabilitation)

Why this matters: Most health systems over-invest in tertiary care (managing advanced disease) and under-invest in primary and secondary prevention. As a resident, you can identify how to shift resources upstream.

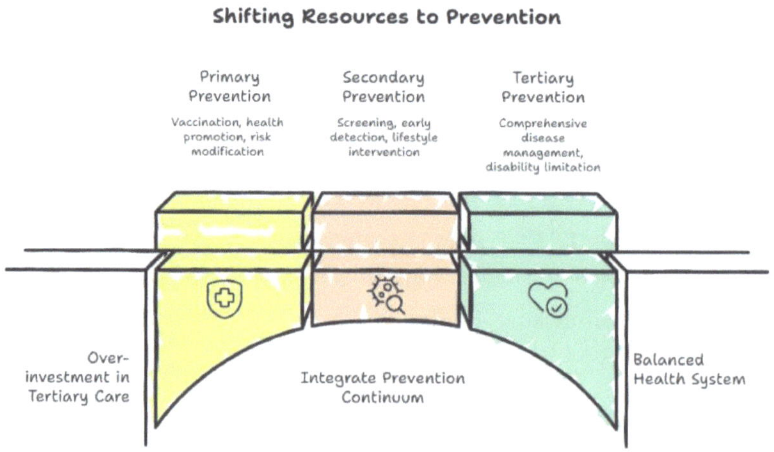

FIGURE *2.1 Shifting resources from over-investment in tertiary care toward balanced primary, secondary, and tertiary prevention.*

Most health systems pour the majority of their resources into **tertiary care**—the expensive, labor-intensive work of managing established disease, treating complications, and responding to crises. This pattern is not accidental; it reflects decades of reimbursement structures, cultural expectations, and organizational habits that reward downstream intervention rather than upstream prevention. Yet this over-investment in late-stage care comes at a profound opportunity cost. Every dollar spent on treating preventable complications is a dollar not spent on preventing disease in the first place.

By contrast, **primary prevention**—intervening before disease develops—and **secondary prevention**—detecting and treating early disease before it progresses—remain chronically underfunded and prioritized. Primary prevention requires long time horizons, cross-sector collaboration, and investments in population health infrastructure that do not yield immediate financial returns. Secondary prevention requires reliable screening systems, data integration, and workflows that identify risk early. Both require organizational commitment to long-term benefit rather than short-term crisis management.

This imbalance creates a persistent and predictable gap: health systems excel at treating advanced disease but struggle to prevent it. For implementation professionals, this gap represents a **recurring, high-leverage opportunity**. Implementation science is uniquely positioned to identify where preventive interventions can be embedded into routine care, how workflows can be redesigned to support earlier action, and which strategies can shift organizational behavior toward upstream investment. This includes mapping where preventive services break down, analyzing variation in screening and follow-up, identifying populations that are systematically missed, and adapting evidence-based preventive interventions to local contexts.

Shifting resources toward earlier prevention is not simply a matter of adding new programs; it requires redesigning systems so that prevention becomes the default rather than the exception. Implementation helps organizations understand their current state, test small changes, evaluate outcomes, and scale what works. In doing so, it enables health systems to move from reactive, crisis-driven care toward proactive, anticipatory models that reduce suffering, improve equity, and ultimately lower costs.

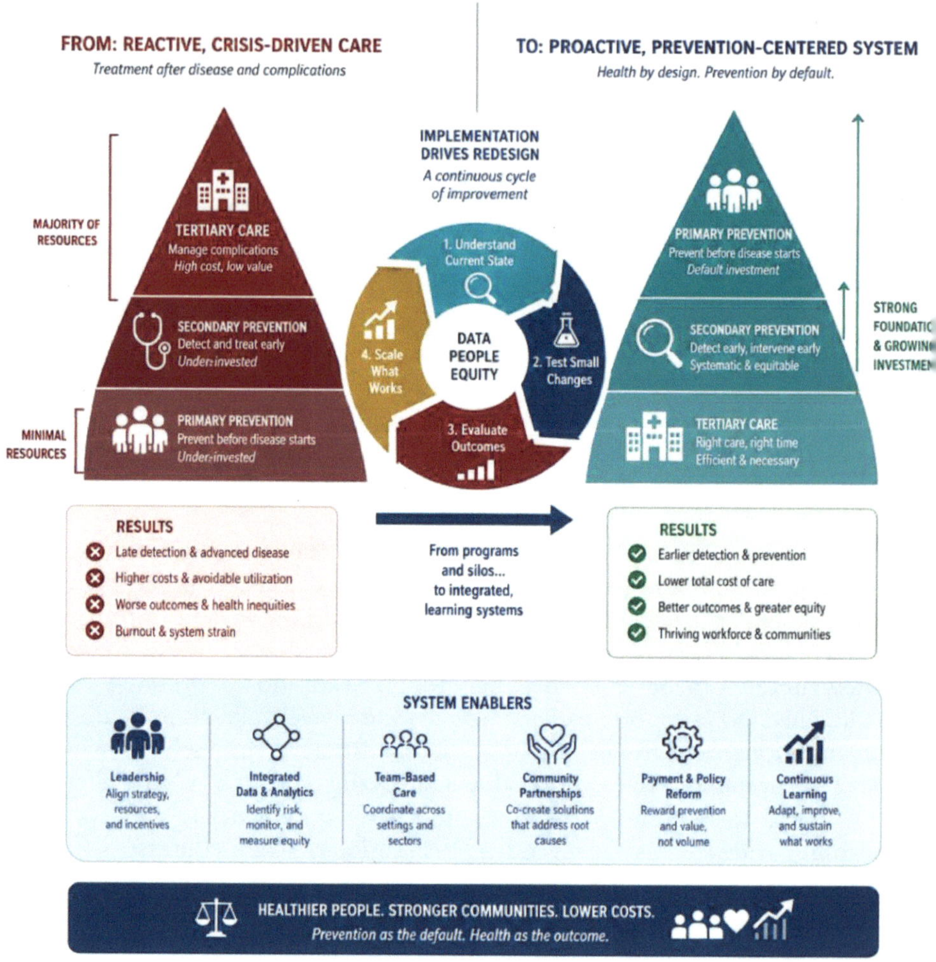
FROM: REACTIVE, CRISIS-DRIVEN CARE
Treatment after disease and complications
TO: PROACTIVE, PREVENTION-CENTERED SYSTEM
Health by design. Prevention by default.
MAJORITY OF RESOURCES
TERTIARY CARE
Manage complications
High cost, low value
SECONDARY PREVENTION
Detect and treat early
Under-invested
MINIMAL RESOURCES
PRIMARY PREVENTION
Prevent before disease starts
Under-invested
IMPLEMENTATION DRIVES REDESIGN
A continuous cycle of improvement
1. Understand Current State
2. Test Small Changes
3. Evaluate Outcomes
4. Scale What Works
DATA PEOPLE EQUITY
PRIMARY PREVENTION
Prevent before disease starts
Default investment
SECONDARY PREVENTION
Detect early, intervene early
Systematic & equitable
TERTIARY CARE
Right care, right time
Efficient & necessary
RESULTS
Late detection & advanced disease
Higher costs & avoidable utilization
Worse outcomes & health inequities
Burnout & system strain
From programs and silos... to integrated, learning systems
RESULTS
Earlier detection & prevention
Lower total cost of care
Better outcomes & greater equity
Thriving workforce & communities
SYSTEM ENABLERS
Leadership
Align strategy, resources, and incentives
Integrated Data & Analytics
Identify risk, monitor, and measure equity
Team-Based Care
Coordinate across settings and sectors
Community Partnerships
Co-create solutions that address root causes
Payment & Policy Reform
Reward prevention and value, not volume
Continuous Learning
Adapt, improve, and sustain what works
HEALTHIER PEOPLE. STRONGER COMMUNITIES. LOWER COSTS.
Prevention as the default. Health as the outcome.

CHAPTER 3

The Composite Regional Academic Health Science Center

3.1 Structure of the Composite AHSC

To anchor the abstract principles of this handbook in a concrete setting, we introduce a composite Regional Academic Health Science Center (AHSC) that serves as the exemplar throughout the volume. The composite institution incorporates features common to contemporary academic medicine.

Components

The composite AHSC comprises:
A flagship tertiary/quaternary hospital providing advanced specialty and subspecialty care, serving as the primary hub for clinical research and innovation. This is where you do most of your inpatient rotations as a resident—the ICUs, ORs, specialty consult services, and complex medical/surgical floors.

A distributed network of ambulatory clinics, including faculty practice sites and community-based primary care centers that serve as training grounds for residents and access points for preventive and chronic care. This is where you see continuity patients, manage chronic diseases, and learn outpatient medicine.

Community health services that extend the reach of the institution into neighborhoods, schools, and non-traditional settings through partnerships with local organizations, public health agencies, and community health centers. This is where you might do community medicine rotations, participate in health fairs, or engage in advocacy work.

A comprehensive suite of residency programs spanning:

- **All primary care disciplines:** Family Medicine, Internal Medicine, Pediatrics
- **Top ten specialty disciplines:** Surgery, Psychiatry, Emergency Medicine, Obstetrics and Gynecology, Neurology, Anesthesiology, Radiology, Pathology, Orthopedics, Dermatology

3.2 The Expanded Mission and Your Role

The contemporary AHSC operates under what is increasingly described as a quintuple mission: patient care, education, research, community collaboration, and health parity. As a resident, you operate simultaneously as patient-care provider, learner, research contributor, and community engager. Your daily work intersects all five missions, and the HSIB provides the conceptual framework to see them not as competing priorities but as integrated dimensions of academic clinical practice.

The composite AHSC operates under a **quadripartite or quintuple mission**: [11-12][14]

1. **Patient care** – Delivering high-quality clinical services.
2. **Education** – Training the next generation of health professionals (that's you)
3. **Research** – Advancing biomedical and health services knowledge.
4. **Community collaboration** – Sustained, bidirectional partnerships with community stakeholders [14-15]
5. **Health parity** – Explicitly addressing disparities and social determinants of health [12][15]

This expanded mission is operationalized through the academic learning health system (aLHS) model, which integrates continuous organizational learning, quality improvement (QI), and the translation of research into practice as embedded features of daily operations. [1] The aLHS is not a static structure but a dynamic ecosystem—a living network that connects clinical care, education, and research through iterative cycles of data generation, reflection, and improvement. It transforms the traditional separation between "doing" and "studying" medicine into a unified process where every clinical encounter contributes to knowledge creation and system advancement.

Within this model, learning is institutionalized. Data from routine care are continuously analyzed to identify gaps, test interventions, and refine processes. Quality improvement becomes a shared responsibility rather than a departmental initiative, and research is no longer confined to academic centers—it is woven into the fabric of everyday practice. The aLHS thus embodies the principle that the best way to improve care is to learn from care itself, creating a feedback loop that accelerates discovery and implementation.

As a senior medical student or resident participating in this system, you occupy a pivotal role at the intersection of learning and practice. You are not merely a trainee acquiring skills; you are an active contributor to the organization's learning cycle. Your daily activities—patient care, documentation, teamwork, and reflection—feed directly into the system's capacity to improve.

Deliver patient care while identifying implementation gaps in real time.

Each clinical encounter becomes an opportunity to observe where evidence-based practices succeed or falter. You learn to recognize patterns—missed screenings, delayed interventions, communication breakdowns—and to translate these observations into actionable improvement goals. This cultivates diagnostic thinking not only about disease but about systems.

Learn through participation in QI projects and implementation initiatives.

You engage in structured improvement cycles such as Plan–Do–Study–Act (PDSA), root-cause analyses, and workflow redesigns. These experiences teach you how to measure change, interpret data, and collaborate across disciplines. You begin to see quality improvement not as abstract exercise but as clinical competency essential to safe, effective care.

Contribute to research by collecting data, testing interventions, and disseminating findings.

In the aLHS, research is democratized. You participate in pragmatic trials, implementation studies, and data-driven evaluations that inform both local practice and broader scholarship. You learn to balance methodological rigor with real-world feasibility, and to communicate findings that advance both science and service.

Engage with communities by understanding social determinants and partnering with patients.

Implementation does not end at the clinic door. You learn to view patients and families as co-designers of care, integrating their perspectives into intervention development and evaluation. This engagement deepens your understanding of equity, cultural responsiveness, and the social context of health, ensuring that system redesigns reflective realities.

Through these experiences, you develop the mindset of a clinician–scientist–improver—someone who sees every process as improvable, every outcome as measurable, and every patient interaction as a source of learning. The aLHS model thus prepares future physicians to lead in environments where evidence generation, implementation, and continuous improvement are inseparable. It operates the vision of a health system that learns from itself, adapts to emerging challenges, and evolves toward higher standards of quality, equity, and efficiency.

CHAPTER 4

How to Design and Execute a Successful QI Project

4.1 The Evidence on Resident QI Education

More than half **than half of U.S. residency programs have implemented QI curricula**, and the evidence shows that QI education combining **didactic instruction with experiential learning** (i.e., you actually do a project, not just read about it) is effective and engaging. [6][16-17]

Residents who complete QI projects report: [6][16][18]

- Increased understanding of QI principles and methods
- Improved confidence in leading improvement efforts
- Greater ability to identify and address systems issues.
- Enhanced collaboration with interdisciplinary teams
- Increased likelihood of pursuing QI work in their careers

Resident-led QI initiatives have demonstrated measurable impact, including:

- Fifty percent reduction in catheter-associated bloodstream infections
- Thirty percent improvement in medication reconciliation accuracy
- Twenty-five percent reduction in door-to-balloon time for STEMI
- Forty percent increase in advance directive completion
- Significant improvements in transitions of care and patient satisfaction

4.2 The Model for Improvement and PDSA Cycles

The Model for Improvement is the most widely taught QI framework. It is organized around three fundamental questions:

1. **What are we trying to accomplish?** (Aim)
2. **How will we know that a change is an improvement?** (Measures)
3. **What changes can we make that will result in improvement?** (Changes)

These questions are operationalized through **Plan-Do-Study-Act (PDSA)** cycles:

- **Plan** – the objective is identified, predictions are made, and the test is planned.
- **Do** – the plan is executed; problems and unexpected observations are documented.
- **Study** – the data are analyzed; the results are compared to the predictions.
- **Act** – modifications are determined; a plan is prepared for the next cycle.

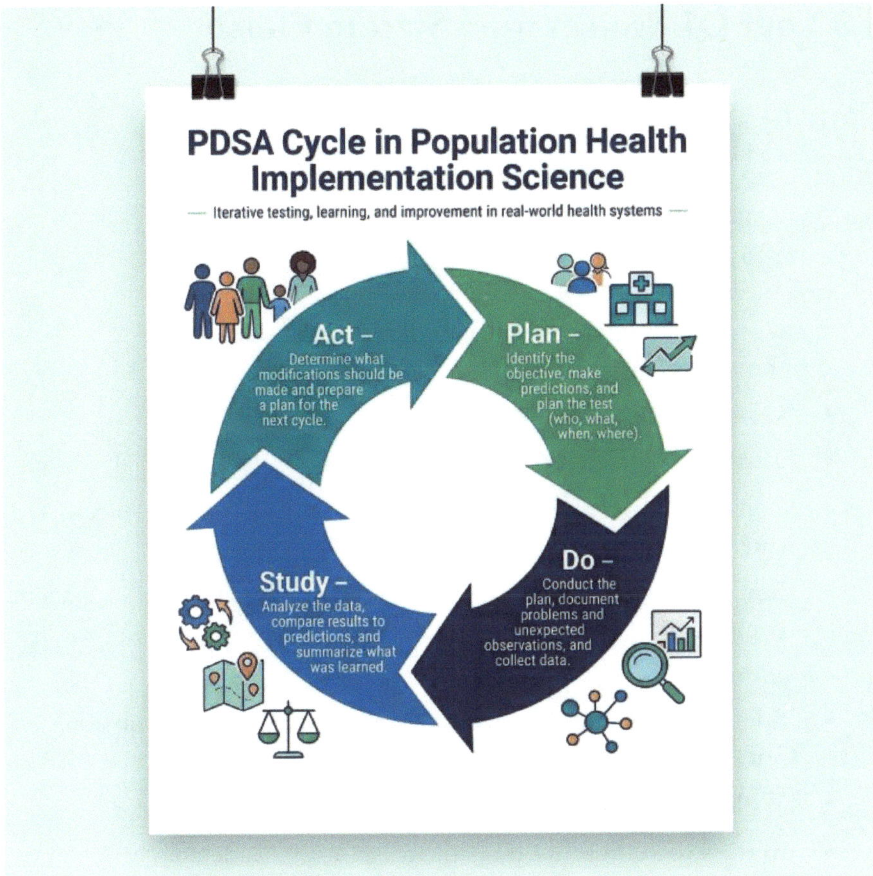

FIGURE *4.1 The PDSA cycle in population-health implementation science.*

A GUIDING PRINCIPLE

Don't try to change the entire hospital on day one. Test your intervention with one patient, one provider, one day. Learn. Adapt. Then scale. The PDSA cycle's value is not theoretical—it is in compressing the learning loop to a size you can run on a Tuesday afternoon.

4.3 Your QI Project from Start to Finish

Step-by-Step Guide: Your QI Project from Start to Finish

Based on successful resident QI curricula, here is a practical 12-week guide: [6][16] [18-19]

Weeks 1-2: Identify and Define the Problem

What to do:

- Observe clinical practice during your rotations.
- Talk to patients, nurses, physicians, pharmacists, and social workers.
- Look for inefficiencies, safety concerns, and gaps in evidence-based care.
- Review institutional data (readmission rates, quality metrics, patient complaints)

How to choose a good problem:

- **Specific and measurable:** "Improve heart failure readmissions" not "Improve quality."
- **Within your scope:** You can influence it as a resident.
- **Maters to stakeholders:** Patients, staff, and leadership care.
- **Evidence-based solutions exist:** You are implementing what works, not inventing from scratch.

Tools to use:

- **Fishbone diagram** (Ishikawa): Identify potential causes of the problem [20]
- **Pareto chart:** Identify 20% of causes responsible for 80% of the problem.
- **Process map:** Visualize the current workflow [20]

Example: You notice that many patients with heart failure are readmitted within 30 days. You review the data and find that your hospital's 30-day HF readmission rate is 28% (the national average is 23%). You talk to patients and learn they do not understand their medications or when to follow up.

Observe clinical practice during your rotations. Talk to patients, nurses, physicians, pharmacists, and social workers. Identify inefficiencies, safety concerns, and gaps in evidence-based care. Review institutional data on readmission rates, quality metrics, and patient complaints. A well-chosen problem is specific, measurable, within your scope as a resident, important to stakeholders, and amenable to evidence-based solutions.

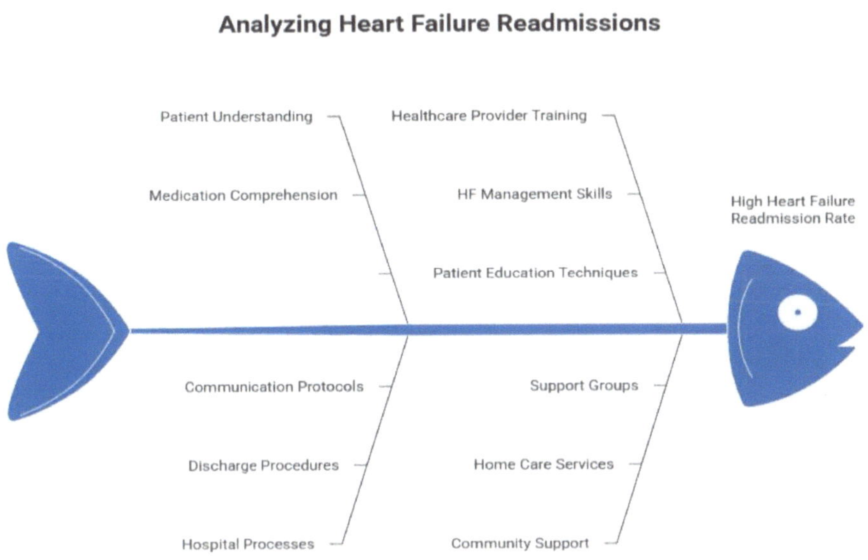

FIGURE *4.2 Fishbone (Ishikawa) diagram for analyzing heart-failure readmissions.*

Weeks 2–3: Understand the Current State

What to do:

- Create a detailed **process map** showing how things currently work [20]
- Collect baseline data on the problem.
- Identify stakeholders (who is affected? who can help? who might resist?)
- Conduct a **root cause analysis** to understand why the problem exists [20]

Stakeholder analysis:

- **Patients:** What barriers do they face?
- **Frontline staff:** What makes their jobs harder?
- **Physicians:** What are their concerns and priorities?
- **Administrators:** What are the financial and regulatory implications?

Example: You map the discharge process and identify gaps: discharge summaries are not sent to PCPs, follow-up appointments are not scheduled before discharge, patients receive written instructions at an eighth-grade reading level, but many have lower health literacy. You conduct a root cause analysis and find that the problem is multifactorial: time pressure, a lack of standardized processes, and poor communication between inpatient and outpatient teams.

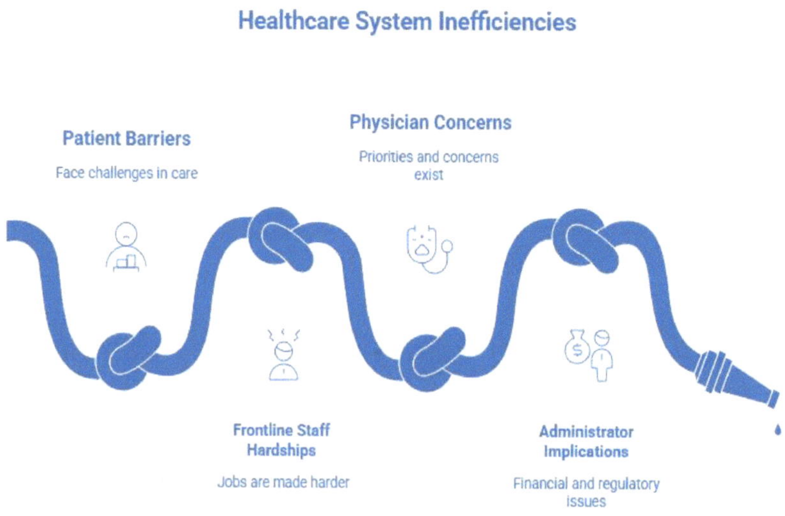

FIGURE *4.3 Healthcare system inefficiencies span patients, frontline staff, physicians, and administrators.*

Weeks 3–4: Search the Evidence and Design the Intervention

What to do:

- Search for **evidence-based interventions** that address similar problems [21-22]
- Use databases: PubMed, Cochrane Library, clinical practice guidelines, AHRQ resources.
- Look for systematic reviews and meta-analyses first (highest level of evidence)
- Appraise the quality of evidence using critical appraisal tools [21]
- Identify best practices from other institutions (benchmarking)

Search strategy:

- Use at least two major databases (e.g., MEDLINE and Epistemonikos) to ensure comprehensive coverage [23-24]
- Use validated search filters (e.g., Clinical Queries) to retrieve relevant systematic reviews [25]
- Check clinical practice guidelines from professional societies (AHA, ACP, ACEP, etc.)

Appraise the evidence:

- Is this a systematic review? Was it done rigorously? (Use AMSTAR-2) [26]
- What is the certainty of evidence? (Understand GRADE ratings) [27]
- Is the intervention feasible in your setting?
- Has it been evaluated in similar populations and settings?

Example: You search PubMed for "heart failure discharge" and "readmission reduction." You found a Cochrane review showing that **structured discharge planning, early follow-up, and patient education reduce 30-day readmissions by 25% (moderate-certainty** evidence). You find AHA guidelines recommending these interventions. You identify a successful program at a similar safety-net hospital

WORKED EXAMPLE: HEART-FAILURE DISCHARGE BUNDLE

Components: Medication reconciliation with teach-back; follow-up appointment scheduled before discharge; patient education materials at low literacy level; 48-hour post-discharge nurse phone call.

Prediction: Reduce 30-day readmission rate from 28% to 20%.

Measurement plan: Clinical outcome – readmission rate. Fidelity – % patients receiving all bundle elements. Acceptability – nurse satisfaction. Sustainability – % sustained at six months.

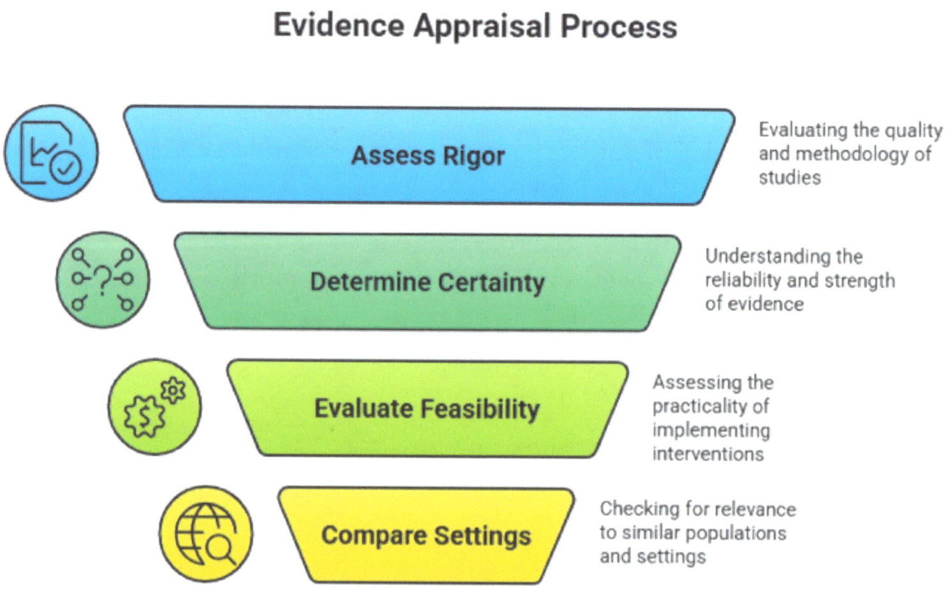

Week 4: Design Your Intervention

What to do:

- Based on evidence and stakeholder input, design a change
- Make it **simple, testable, and adaptable.**
- Predict what will happen when you implement the change.
- Plan how you will measure success (clinical outcomes + implementation outcomes)

Key principles:

- **Adapt, do not adopt:** Tailor the evidence-based intervention to your local context.
- **Address barriers:** If time is a barrier, build the intervention into the existing workflow.
- **Engage stakeholders:** Get buy-in from nurses, attendings, case managers, and patients.
- **Plan for sustainability:** How will this continue after you rotate off service?

Example: You design a **heart failure discharge bundle** that includes:

1. Medication reconciliation with teach-back.
2. Follow-up appointment scheduled before discharge
3. Patient education using low-literacy materials.
4. Phone call from nurse within 48 hours of discharge.

You predict this will reduce 30-day readmissions from 28% to 20%. Your plan to measure:

- **Clinical outcome:** 30-day readmission rate
- **Implementation outcomes:** % of patients who receive all bundle elements (fidelity), nurse satisfaction with bundle (acceptability), % sustained at 6 months (sustainability)

Weeks 5-8: Implement PDSA Cycles

What to do:

- Start with a **small-scale test** (e.g., five patients, 1 week, one team)
- Collect data during the test.
- Analyze results and compare predictions.
- Modify the intervention based on what you learned.
- Repeat with progressively larger tests.

PDSA Cycle 1 (Week 5):

- **Plan:** Test discharge bundle with 5 HF patients on your team this week
- **Do:** Residents complete bundle for five patients; document time required and barriers encountered
- **Study:** 4 of 5 patients received all bundle elements; average time 20 minutes; nurses report bundle is acceptable, but discharge summary template needs revision
- **Act:** Revise discharge summary template; plan to evaluate with fifteen patients' next cycle

PDSA Cycle 2 (Week 6):

- **Plan:** Test revised bundle with 15 HF patients across two teams
- **Do:** Implement revised bundle
- **Study:** 12 of 15 patients received all elements (80%); three patients did not get a follow-up schedule because the clinic was full
- **Act:** Work with the clinic to create dedicated post-discharge HF slots; plan to expand to all HF discharges

PDSA Cycle 3 (Weeks 7-8):

- **Plan:** Implement bundle for all HF discharges on medicine service (approximately thirty patients)
- **Do:** All teams use bundle
- **Study:** 25 of 30 patients received all elements (83%); readmission rate for these patients is 18% (vs. 28% baseline)
- **Act:** Present results to hospital QI committee; propose hospital-wide implementation

Weeks 9-10: Analyze and Present Results

What to do:

- Create **run charts** or **statistical process control (SPC) charts** to display data over time.
- Calculate the impact of your intervention (absolute and relative risk reduction, number needed to treat)
- Prepare a poster or presentation for stakeholders.
- Discuss sustainability: How can this change be maintained?
- Identify lessons learned and next steps.

Data visualization:

- **Run chart:** Plot your outcome measure over time with a median line; look for shifts, trends, or runs [19]
- **SPC chart:** Add control limits to identify special cause vs. common cause variation.
- **Before-and-after comparison:** Compare baseline period to intervention period.

Example results:

- Baseline 30-day readmission rate: 28% (42 of 150 patients)
- Intervention period readmission rate: 18% (27 of 150 patients)
- Absolute risk reduction: ten percentage points
- Relative risk reduction: 36%
- Number needed to treat: 10 (for every ten patients who receive the bundle, one readmission is prevented)

Sustainability plan:

- Integrate bundle into EHR as a required discharge checklist.
- Train all residents and nurses in bundle use
- Assign a nurse champion to monitor compliance.
- Present results at departmental QI meeting and grand rounds
- Submit abstract to regional or national QI conference.

Week 11-12: Disseminate and Sustain

What to do:

- Present your project at hospital QI meetings, grand rounds, or residency conference.
- Submit abstract to regional or national conference (SHM, ACP, ACEP, etc.)
- Write up your project for publication (many journals publish QI work: BMJ Quality & Safety, Joint Commission Journal on Quality and Patient Safety, American Journal of Medical Quality)
- Work with hospital leadership to integrate your intervention into standard practice.
- Hand off to a sustainability team (QI department, nursing leadership, etc.)

Dissemination venues:

- Hospital QI committee
- Departmental grand rounds
- Residency research day
- Regional QI collaborative (e.g., Michigan Hospital Medicine Safety Consortium)
- National conferences (SHM, ACP, ACEP, AAFP, AAP, etc.)
- Peer-reviewed journals

4.4 Common Tools and When to Use Them

TABLE 4.1 Principal QI tools and their application

Tool	Purpose	When to Use	How to Use	References
Process Map	Visualize current workflow	Under-standing the current state	Map each step from start to finish; identify delays, handoffs, and decision points	[1]
Fishbone Diagram	Identify root causes	Problem diagnosis	Organize causes into categories (people, process, equipment, environ-ment, etc.)	[1]
Pareto Chart	Prioritize problems	Deciding what to tackle first	Rank causes by frequency; focus on the vital few	[1]

Tool	Purpose	When to Use	How to Use	Reference s
Driver Diagram	Map factors contrib-uting to aim	Planning interven-tions	Identify primary and secondary drivers; link to specific interven-tions	[2]
PDSA Cycle	Evaluate changes on a small scale	Implementi ng and refining	Plan-Do-Study-Act; start small, learn, adapt, scale	[2-4]
Run Chart	Display data over time	Monitoring improve-ment	Plot outcome measure over time; look for shifts and trends	[4]
Control Chart (SPC)	Distin-guish signal from noise	Determin-ing if change is real	Add control limits to run chart; identify special cause variation	[4]

Tool	Purpose	When to Use	How to Use	Reference s
Stake-holder Analysis	Identify who to engage	Engage-ment planning	Map stakehold-ers by influence and interest; develop engage-ment strategies	[5]

[5] [16-17] [19-20]

CHAPTER 5

Evidence-Based Medicine Skills for Implementation

5.1 The Five Steps of EBM in Clinical Practice

The Sicily Statement defines five steps of evidence-based medicine:
As a resident, you use evidence-based medicine (EBM) skills daily. The **Sicily Statement** defines five steps: [1]

1. **Ask** – Formulate answerable clinical questions using PICO (Patient, Intervention, Comparison, Outcome)
2. **Acquire** – Search for the best available evidence efficiently.
3. **Appraise** – Critically evaluate the evidence for validity and applicability.
4. **Apply** – Integrate evidence with clinical expertise and patient values.
5. **Assess** – Evaluate the outcomes of the decision.

For implementation projects, you use the same skills:

Ask: "What interventions reduce heart failure readmissions in safety-net hospitals?"
Acquire: Search PubMed, Cochrane, AHRQ; find systematic reviews and guidelines
Appraise: Assess the quality of evidence using GRADE; determine if interventions are feasible in your setting
Apply: Adapt the evidence-based intervention to your local context, engaging stakeholders
Assess: Measure clinical outcomes (readmissions) and implementation outcomes (adoption, fidelity, sustainability)

Table 5.1 Comparison of systems used to assess evidence

	Classification system[a]					
	ACC/AHA	AHRQ	GRADE	NICE	OCEBM	USPSTF
Terminology	Level/quality of evidence	Strength of evidence	Certainty/quality of evidence	Quality of evidence	Levels of evidence	Quality of the overall evidence
Considerations	Study design, No. of studies, consistency with indirect evidence	Study design, applicability, inconsistency	Risk of bias, inconsistency, imprecision, indirectness, publication bias, magnitude of effect, dose-response relationship, opposing residual confounding	Risk of bias, inconsistency, imprecision, indirectness, publication bias	Study design, effect size, sample size, risk of bias	Risk of bias, applicability, inconsistency, No. of studies/participants
Levels	A, B-R (randomized), B-NR (nonrandomized), C-LD (limited data), C-EO (expert opinion)	High, moderate, low, insufficient	High, moderate, low, very low	High, moderate, low, very low	Levels 1-5	Good, fair, poor

Abbreviations: ACC/AHA, American College of Cardiology/American Heart Association; AHRQ, Agency for Healthcare Research and Quality; GRADE, Grading of Recommendations Assessment, Development and Evaluation; NICE, National Institute for Health and Care Excellence; OCEBM, Oxford Centre for Evidence-Based Medicine; USPSTF, US Preventive Services Task Force.

[a] Discrepancies in the numbers of systems exist between Tables 1 and 2 because the AHRQ and OCEBM do not have a system for classifying the strength of recommendations.

Source: How to Interpret and Use a Clinical Practice Guideline or Recommendation: Users' Guides to Medical Literature.

5.2 Asking the Right Question: PICO for Implementation

The PICO framework helps you formulate focused, answerable questions: [1-2]
P – Patient/Population: Who are you trying to help?
I – Intervention: What are you considering doing?
C – Comparison: What is the alternative (usual care, another intervention, or nothing)?
O – Outcome: What are you trying to accomplish?

Clinical example:

- **P:** Adults with heart failure discharged from a safety-net hospital
- **I:** Structured discharge bundle (medication reconciliation, follow-up scheduling, patient education, post-discharge phone call)
- **C:** Usual discharge care
- **O:** 30-day all-cause readmission rate

PICO question: "In adults with heart failure discharged from a safety-net hospital, does a structured discharge bundle compared to usual care reduce 30-day all-cause readmissions?"

For implementation questions, you can extend PICO to PICOTS:
T – Timing: When should the intervention be delivered? (e.g., within 48 hours of discharge)
S – Setting: Where will it be implemented? (e.g., urban safety-net hospital)
Implementation-focused PICO example:

- **P:** Internal medicine residents
- **I:** Structured QI curriculum with experiential learning (doing a project)
- **C:** Didactic lectures alone
- **O:** Confidence in leading QI initiatives, knowledge of QI methods

PICO question: "In internal medicine residents, does a structured QI curriculum with experiential learning compared to didactic lectures alone improve confidence and knowledge in leading QI initiatives?"

5.3 Acquiring Evidence: Where and How to Search

The hierarchy of evidence applicable to implementation work runs, in approximate order of authority, from clinical practice guidelines through systematic reviews and meta-analyses, implementation-science studies, quality-improvement reports from comparable institutions, and finally expert consensus statements. The optimal search strategy combines MEDLINE and Epistemonikos with reference checking, achieving recall above 98%.

The hierarchy of evidence for implementation:

1. **Clinical practice guidelines** from professional societies (AHA, ACC, ACP, ACEP, ACOG, AAP, etc.)
2. **Systematic reviews and meta-analyses** (Cochrane Library, AHRQ Evidence Reports)
3. **Implementation of science studies** (pragmatic trials, hybrid effectiveness-implementation trials)

4. **Quality improvement reports** from similar institutions
5. **Expert consensus statements**

Where to search:

Resource	What It Offers	When to Use	URL
PubMed/MEDLINE	Comprehensive biomedical literature	First-line search for any clinical question	pubmed.ncbi.nlm.nih.gov
Cochrane Library	High-quality systematic reviews	Finding synthesized evidence on interventions	Cochranelibrary.com
Epistemonikos	Database of systematic reviews	Comprehensive search for reviews	epistemonikos.org
AHRQ Evidence Reports	Systematic reviews on effectiveness and implementation	Finding evidence on health services interventions	Effectivehealthcare.ahrq.gov
Guidelines International Network	Clinical practice guidelines	Finding authoritative recommendations	g-i-n.net

Resource	What It Offers	When to Use	URL
National Guideline Clearing-house	U.S. clinical practice guidelines	Finding specialty-specific guidelines	guideline.gov (archived; use society websites)
UpToDate/ DynaMed	Point-of-care clinical sum-maries	Quick clinical questions during patient care	Institutional subscription
Google Scholar	Broad aca-demic search	Finding grey lit-erature, conference abstracts	scholar.google.com

[1-5]

Search strategy for implementation projects:

Step 1: Start with clinical practice guidelines.

- Search the website of the relevant professional society (e.g., American Heart Association for heart failure)
- Look for "Clinical Practice Guidelines" or "Scientific Statements."
- Check the strength of recommendations and quality of evidence.

Step 2: Search for systematic reviews

- Use PubMed Clinical Queries filter for "Systematic Reviews."
- Search for Cochrane Library and Epistemonikos
- Use search terms: [condition] AND [intervention] AND ("systematic review" OR "meta-analysis")

Example search: "heart failure" AND "discharge planning" AND "systematic review"

Step 3: Search for implementation studies

- Add implementation-focused terms to your search: "implementation" OR "quality improvement" OR "pragmatic trial" OR "real-world."
- Look for studies in settings similar to yours (safety-net hospitals, academic medical centers, community hospitals)

Step 4: Check for local or regional QI collaboratives

- Michigan Hospital Medicine Safety Consortium
- California Maternal Quality Care Collaborative
- Vermont Oxford Network (neonatal care)
- Institute for Healthcare Improvement (IHI) resources

Validated search strategy:
Research shows that searching **both MEDLINE and Epistemonikos**, supplemented by reference checking, yields the highest recall for systematic reviews in biomedical topics, with inclusion rates exceeding 98% and approaching 99.6% when accounting for geographic publication biases. [3-4] The American Heart Association recommends expanding searches to include additional databases and grey literature as appropriate for the clinical question. [6]

Time-saving tips for busy residents:

- **Use Clinical Queries filters** in PubMed to retrieve relevant systematic reviews with high sensitivity and specificity [5]
- **Start with UpToDate or DynaMed** for a quick overview, then dig deeper into primary sources.
- **Set up PubMed alerts** for your topic to receive new publications automatically.
- **Use reference management software** (Zotero, Mendeley, EndNote) to organize your search results.

5.4 Appraising Evidence: Is It Valid and Applicable?

Three questions guide critical appraisal: Is the evidence valid? (internal validity). Is it applicable? (external validity). Is it important? (clinical significance). Specialized tools include AMSTAR-2 for systematic reviews, GRADE for certainty of evidence, and AGREE II for clinical practice guidelines.

Once you have found evidence, you need to critically appraise it. The key questions are: [2] [7-9]

Is the evidence valid? (Internal validity: Can I trust the results?)

Is the evidence applicable? (External validity: Does it apply to my patients and setting?)

Is the evidence important? (Clinical significance: Will it make a meaningful difference?)

Appraising systematic reviews:

Use the **AMSTAR-2 tool** (A MeaSurement Tool to Assess systematic Reviews) to assess quality: [9]

Critical domains:

1. Did the review include a PICO question and inclusion criteria?
2. Did the search strategy include at least two databases?
3. Did reviewers perform study selection and data extraction in duplicate?
4. Did reviewers assess risk of bias in included studies?
5. Did reviewers use appropriate methods for meta-analysis?
6. Did reviewers consider risk of bias when interpreting results?
7. Did reviewers assess publication bias?

Quick appraisal questions:

- Is this a systematic review or just a narrative review? (Systematic reviews use explicit, reproducible methods)
- Did they search multiple databases? (At least MEDLINE + one other) [3-4][8]
- Did they assess study quality/risk of bias? (Using tools like Cochrane ROB-2, ROBINS-I) [9]
- Did they use GRADE to rate certainty of evidence? [6-7]

Understanding GRADE (Grading of Recommendations Assessment, Development and Evaluation):

GRADE rates the **certainty of evidence** as: [6-7]

- **High:** We are noticeably confident that the true effect lies close to the estimate
- **Moderate:** We are moderately confident; the true effect is close to the estimate, but there is a possibility it is different
- **Low:** Our confidence is limited; the true effect may be different from the estimate
- **Exceptionally low:** We have extraordinarily little confidence; the true effect is different from the estimate.

Factors that lower certainty:

- Risk of bias (study limitations)
- Inconsistency (unexplained heterogeneity)
- Indirectness (differences in population, intervention, or outcomes)
- Imprecision (wide confidence intervals, small sample sizes)
- Publication bias

Factors that raise certainty:

- Large magnitude of effect
- Dose-response gradient.
- All plausible confounding would reduce the effect.

Comparing evidence rating systems:

Different organizations use different systems to rate evidence. The table below, from Brignardello-Petersen et al., published in JAMA, illustrates how organizations such as the American College of Cardiology/American

Heart Association, the US Preventive Services Task Force, and the Agency for Healthcare Research and Quality classify the certainty of evidence. [7] Understanding these systems helps you interpret guidelines and apply them appropriately in your implementation projects.

Appraising clinical practice guidelines:

Use the **AGREE II tool** (Appraisal of Guidelines for Research & Evaluation) to assess guideline quality: [10]

Key domains:

1. **Scope and purpose:** Are the objectives clearly described?
2. **Stakeholder involvement:** Were patients and target users involved?
3. **Rigor of development:** Was the search systematic? Was evidence appraised? Were recommendations linked to evidence?
4. **Clarity of presentation:** Are recommendations specific and unambiguous?
5. **Applicability:** Are barriers to implementation discussed? Are resource implications considered?
6. **Editorial independence:** Is the guideline free from conflicts of interest?

Quick appraisal questions for guidelines:

- Is this from a reputable professional society?
- Is it current? (Guidelines >5 years old may be outdated)
- Are recommendations graded by strength and quality of evidence?
- Are conflicts of interest disclosed?
- Does it address implementation barriers?

Appraising implementation studies:

For implementation of science studies, ask: [11-12]

Was the implementation strategy clearly described?

- Can you replicate it in your setting?
- What were the active ingredients?

Were implementation outcomes measured?

- Adoption, fidelity, acceptability, feasibility, sustainability, cost?

Was the context described?

- Setting characteristics (urban/rural, academic/community, resource level)
- Population characteristics (demographics, socioeconomic status, health literacy)
- Organizational characteristics (culture, leadership, readiness for change)

Were barriers and facilitators identified?

- What made implementation succeed or fail?
- Are these barriers present in your setting?

Were equity considerations addressed?

- Did the intervention reach underserved populations?
- Were there differential effects by race, ethnicity, language, insurance status?

5.5 Applying Evidence: Adaptation to Local Context

Evidence rarely transfers directly from one setting to another. Effective implementation requires adaptation to the local context while maintaining fidelity to the core components that produce the intervention's effects. The CFIR framework organizes contextual assessment across five domains: intervention characteristics, outer setting, inner setting, characteristics of individuals, and process.

The adaptation process:

Step 1: Identify core components.

- What are the essential elements that cannot be changed without losing effectiveness?
- Example: For a heart failure discharge bundle, core components are medication reconciliation, follow-up scheduling, and patient education

Step 2: Identify adaptable periphery.

- What can be modified to fit your setting?
- Example: The format of patient education materials (video vs. written), the timing of follow-up calls (24 vs. 48 hours), who delivers the intervention (nurse vs. pharmacist vs. resident)

Step 3: Assess local barriers and facilitators.

Use a framework like **CFIR (Consolidated Framework for Implementation Research)** to systematically assess your context: [11][14]

CFIR domains:

1. **Intervention characteristics:** Complexity, adaptability, cost, evidence strength
2. **Outer setting:** Patient needs, external policies, peer pressure
3. **Inner setting:** Structural characteristics, culture, readiness for change, resources
4. **Characteristics of individuals:** Knowledge, beliefs, self-efficacy, stage of change
5. **Process:** Planning, engaging, executing, reflecting & evaluating

Practical assessment questions:

- **Intervention:** Is it too complex for our workflow? Can we simplify it?
- **Outer setting:** Do payers reimburse this? What do patients want?
- **Inner setting:** Do we have the resources (staff, time, technology)? Is leadership supportive?
- **Individuals:** Do staff have the skills? Are they motivated? What are their concerns?
- **Process:** Who will champion this? How will we engage stakeholders? What is the timeline?

Step 4: Engage stakeholders in adaptation.

- **Frontline staff:** "What would make this work in your workflow?"
- **Patients:** "What barriers would prevent you from participating?"
- **Leadership:** "What resources can you commit? What outcomes matter most?"

- **IT/informatics:** "How can we build this into the EHR?"

Step 5: Document your adaptations.

- Keep a log of what you changed and why.
- Distinguish between **fidelity-consistent adaptations** (maintain core components) and **fidelity-inconsistent adaptations** (alter core components)
- This will help you interpret your results and share lessons learned.

Example: **Adapting a heart failure discharge bundle**

Evidence-based intervention from literature:

- Medication reconciliation by pharmacist
- Follow-up appointment within 7 days
- Patient education is using teach-back method.
- Home visit by nurse within 48 hours

Your local context:

- Safety-net hospital with limited pharmacy resources
- Outpatient clinics are often booked for 2-3 weeks out.
- No home health nursing available for all patients
- Residents rotate every 4 weeks.

Your adapted intervention:

- **Core component maintained:** Medication reconciliation (adapted: done by resident with pharmacist consultation for complex cases)
- **Core component maintained:** Follow-up appointment (adapted: within 7-10 days; created dedicated post-discharge slots)
- **Core component maintained:** Patient education with teach-back (adapted: used low-literacy materials in multiple languages)
- **Peripheral component adapted:** Phone call instead of home visit within 48 hours (more feasible; still maintains contact)
- **New component added:** Resident handoff tool to ensure continuity across rotations.

5.6 Assessing Outcomes: Did It Work?

The final step is evaluating whether implementation succeeded. Both clinical outcomes (did patients improve?) and implementation outcomes (was the intervention adopted and sustained?) are measured. Analysis distinguishes failure of the intervention from failure of implementation: if fidelity was low, the problem is implementation, not the intervention itself.

Clinical outcomes answer: "Did patients get better?"

- Readmission rates
- Mortality
- Disease control (HbA1c, blood pressure, LDL)
- Patient-reported outcomes (quality of life, symptom burden)
- Safety outcomes (adverse events, complications)

Implementation outcomes answer: "Was the intervention adopted and sustained?" [11-12]

- **Reach:** What percentage of eligible patients received the intervention?
- **Adoption:** What percentage of eligible providers/sites used it?
- **Fidelity:** Was it delivered as intended?
- **Acceptability:** Did stakeholders find it acceptable?
- **Feasibility:** Could it be delivered through routine practice?
- **Sustainability:** Was it maintained over time?
- **Cost:** What were the resource requirements?

Choosing the right measures:

For your QI project, select:

- **1-2 clinical outcome measures** that matter to patients and align with organizational priorities.
- **2-3 implementation outcome measures** that will help you understand why the intervention succeeded or failed.
- **1-2 balancing measures** to detect unintended consequences.
- **1-2 process measures** to monitor implementation in real time.

Example measurement plan for heart failure discharge bundle: [11-12] [15-16]

Measure Type	Specific Measure	Data Source	Target
Clinical Outcome	30-day all-cause readmission rate	EHR/ administrative data	Reduce from 28% to 20%
Clinical Outcome	7-day post-discharge follow-up rate	EHR	Increase from 60% to 85%
Implementation Outcome	% of eligible patients who receive bundle	Manual chart review	≥80%
Implementation Outcome	Fidelity % of bundle components completed	Discharge checklist	≥4 of 5 components for ≥80% of patients
Implementation Outcome	Acceptability: Nurse satisfaction	Survey (1-5 scale)	Mean ≥4.0

Measure Type	Specific Measure	Data Source	Target
Balancing Measure	Length of stay	EHR	No increase
Balancing Measure	Time to discharge	EHR	No increase >30 minutes
Process Measure	% of patients with medication reconciliation completed	EHR	100%
Process Measure	% of patients with follow-up scheduled at discharge	EHR	≥85%

Data collection strategies:

Use existing data when possible:

- EHR reports (readmissions, follow-up visits, lab values)
- Administrative data (length of stay, costs)
- Quality dashboards (core measures, patient satisfaction)

Collect new data only when necessary:

- Manual chart review (use standardized abstraction forms)
- Surveys (keep them short; use validated instruments when available)
- Direct observation (time-motion studies, fidelity checklists)

Keep the data collection burden low:

- Integrate data collection into workflow (e.g., discharge checklist that also serves as data collection tool)
- Use sampling if reviewing all charts is not feasible (e.g., review twenty charts per month)
- Automate when possible (EHR reports, REDCap surveys)

Analyzing your data:

For running charts and control charts: [16]

- Plot your outcome measure over time.
- Look for **shifts** (6 or more consecutive points above or below the median)
- Look for **trends** (5 or more consecutive points all increasing or all decreasing)
- Look for **runs** (unusually long sequences on one side of the media)
- These patterns suggest that your intervention caused a real change (not just random variation)

For before-and-after comparisons:

- Calculate **absolute risk reduction:** (Baseline rate) - (Intervention rate)
    - Example: 28% - 18% = 10 percentage points
- Calculate **relative risk reduction:** (Absolute risk reduction) / (Baseline rate)
    - Example: 10% / 28% = 36% relative reduction
- Calculation **number needed to treat (NNT):** 1 / (Absolute risk reduction)
    - Example: 1 / 0.10 = 10 (for every 10 patients who receive the bundle, 1 readmission is prevented)

For statistical significance:

- If you have a statistician or epidemiologist available, consult them.
- Common tests: Chi-square for categorical outcomes, t-test for continuous outcomes, interrupted time series analysis for longitudinal data
- Remember: **Statistical significance ≠ clinical significance.** A minor change that is statistically significant may not be meaningful to patients or worth the resources required.

Interpreting your results:

If your intervention worked:

- What were the key success factors?
- Can you sustain it? Scale it to other units or sites.
- What were the costs and benefits?
- Were there unintended consequences (positive or negative)?

If your intervention did not work:

- Was it a failure of the intervention (the evidence-based practice does not work in your setting) or a failure of implementation (you could not deliver it as intended)?
- Check your fidelity data: If fidelity was low, the problem is implementation, not the intervention.
- What were the barriers? Can they be addressed?
- Should you try a different intervention, or modify your implementation strategy?

If results were mixed:

- Did the intervention work for some patients but not others? (Examine subgroup analyses by age, race, ethnicity, insurance, and health literacy)
- Did some sites or providers succeed while others did not? (Identify best practices from high performers)
- Were some components of the intervention effective while others were not? (Consider simplifying or focusing on high-yield elements)

5.7 Effective Strategies for Learning and Applying EBM

Evidence-based medicine is best learned in clinical settings where the skills can be applied to real patients.

Research on EBM education identifies several effective strategies for residents: [1-2] [17-18]

Clinically integrated teaching and learning – EBM is best learned in clinical settings where you can apply skills to real patients. [19] Successful implementation requires partnerships between core EBM teams, clinical faculty, and frontline clinicians. [19]

Practical tips:

- During rounds, when a clinical question arises, it takes 5 minutes to search for evidence on your phone or tablet.
- Use the "EBM teaching script": Ask → Acquire → Appraise → Apply → Assess.
- Keep a log of clinical questions and the evidence you found; review it weekly.

Multifaceted curricula – Combining lectures, workshops, online modules, and firsthand practice is more effective than any single method. [17]

Practical tips:

- Complete online modules (e.g., Institute for Healthcare Improvement Open School, Cochrane Interactive Learning)
- Attend EBM or QI workshops at your institution or national conferences.
- Practice critical appraisal using journal clubs.
- Apply skills in your QI project.

Four Component Instructional Design (4C/ID) model – To facilitate transfer of EBM skills from classroom to clinical practice, training should include: [18]

1. **Learning tasks:** Authentic, whole-task practice (e.g., answering a clinical question from start to finish)
2. **Supportive information:** Conceptual knowledge (e.g., study designs, bias, GRADE)
3. **Procedural information:** Step-by-step guidance (e.g., how to search PubMed, how to calculate NNT)
4. **Part-task practice:** Repetition of specific skills (e.g., practicing PICO questions, practicing critical appraisal)

Practical tips:

- **Whole-task practice:** During your QI project, you will go through the entire EBM process from question formulation to outcome assessment.
- **Supportive information:** Review study design and biostatistics resources (e.g., JAMA Users' Guides to Medical Literature) [7]
- **Procedural information:** Use checklists and templates (PICO worksheet, critical appraisal checklist, search strategy template)
- **Part-task practice:** Set aside time each week to practice one skill (e.g., Monday: practice PICO questions; Wednesday: practice searching; Friday: practice critical appraisal)

Assessment using validated tools – The **Fresno test** is a validated 212-point assessment of EBM knowledge and skills. Studies show significant improvements in Fresno scores following multifaceted EBM curricula (an average increase of 38.7 marks; $p < 0.001$). [17]

Practical tips:

- Take a baseline Fresno test at the start of your residency.
- Retake it after completing your QI project or EBM curriculum.
- Use your score to identify areas for improvement (e.g., if you score low on critical appraisal, focus on that skill)

Resources for learning EBM:

Resource	What It Offers	Access
JAMA Users' Guides to the Medical Literature	Comprehensive EBM textbook and article series	jamaevidence.com or PubMed
Cochrane Interactive Learning	Free online EBM training modules	training.cochrane.org
IHI Open School	Free QI and patient safety courses (certificates available)	ihi.org/education/IHIOpenSchool
Center for Evidence-Based Medicine (Oxford)	Critical appraisal tools, calculators, tutorials	cebm.net
McMaster PLUS	Evidence summaries and alerts	mcmasterplus.com
Essential Evidence Plus	Point-of-care summaries, calculators, decision aids	essentialevidenceplus.com
PubMed Clinical Queries	Pre-filtered searches for clinical questions	ncbi.nlm.nih.gov/pubmed/clinical

[1-2][5][7][17]

Key Takeaways for Section 5:

✓ **EBM skills are essential for the implementation of science.** The same five steps (Ask, Acquire, Appraise, Apply, Assess) apply to both clinical questions and implementation projects.

✓ **Use PICO to formulate focused questions.** This makes your literature search more efficient and your project more focused.

✓ **Search systematically.** Use at least two databases (MEDLINE + Epistemonikos), start with systematic reviews and guidelines, and use validated search filters. [3-5]

✓ **Appraise critically.** Not all evidence is created equal. Use tools like AMSTAR-2 for systematic reviews and AGREE II for guidelines. [9-10]

✓ **Understand GRADE.** Knowing the certainty of evidence helps you make informed decisions about which interventions to implement. [6-7]

✓ **Adapt, do not just adopt.** Tailor evidence-based interventions to your local context while maintaining fidelity to core components. [11][13]

✓ **Measure both clinical and implementation outcomes.** Success is not just "Did patients improve?" but also "Was the intervention adopted, delivered with fidelity, and sustained?" [11-12]

✓ **Learn by doing.** The best way to develop EBM skills is to apply them to real clinical questions and QI projects in your daily practice. [18-19]

CHAPTER 6

Population Health and Biopsychosocial Determinants of Health

6.1 The Biopsychosocial Model: Beyond the Biomedical

The **biopsychosocial model (BPSM)**, as proposed by George Engel in 1977, is an improvement over the biomedical model, considering psychological, social, and biological factors relevant to health and disease. [1-2] Over the past few decades, substantial evidence has accumulated supporting the BPSM, and it is now the basis of the World Health Organization's International Classification of Functioning (WHO ICF) and is used to structure clinical guidelines. [3]

Why the biopsychosocial model matters for clinicians:
Chronic diseases now account for most morbidity and many deaths in Western countries. Healthcare systems designed around acute biomedical care models are struggling to improve patient-reported outcomes and reduce healthcare costs. [3] The biopsychosocial model provides a framework for understanding and addressing the complex, interacting factors that drive chronic disease.

The BPSM accommodates psychological, social, and biological treatment effects. Personal, interpersonal, and institutional aspects of clinical care—often assigned to the "art" of healthcare rather than the science—can be accommodated and theorized in the BPSM. [1]

The BPSM enables patient-centered care. Through this model, physicians can understand patients in their context, aiding the development of tailored, individualized treatment plans that consider relevant biological, psychological, and socio-cultural-spiritual factors affecting health and longitudinal care. [4]

The BPS-Pathways Model:
Recent work has refined the biopsychosocial model into a more testable framework. The **BPS-Pathways model** presents all six potential pathways among biological (B), psychological (P), and social (S) factors: [5-6]

- **S→P pathway:** Social factors (e.g., social support, discrimination, socioeconomic status) influence psychological factors (e.g., stress, coping, self-efficacy)
- **B→P pathway:** Biological factors (e.g., chronic pain, fatigue, hormonal changes) influence psychological factors.
- **P→B pathway:** Psychological factors (e.g., chronic stress, depression, health behaviors) influence biological outcomes.
- **S→B pathway:** Social factors directly influence biology (often mediated by psychological factors)
- **PS pathway:** Psychological factors influence social functioning and relationships.
- **B→S pathway:** Biological factors (e.g., disability, illness) influence social participation.

Clinical application: When caring for a patient with poorly controlled diabetes, consider:

- **Biological:** Insulin resistance, beta-cell dysfunction, comorbidities
- **Psychological:** Depression (present in 20-30% of diabetics), health beliefs, self-efficacy, coping strategies
- **Social:** Food insecurity, housing instability, social support, health literacy, access to care, neighborhood environment

An intervention that addresses only the biological factors (e.g., adding another medication) may fail if the patient cannot afford the medication (social), does not believe it will help (psychological), or is too depressed to take it consistently (psychological).

6.2 Population Health: Definitions and Distinctions

Population health is defined as "the health outcomes of a group of individuals, including the distribution of such outcomes within the group," and the field of population health includes health outcomes, patterns of health determinants, and policies and interventions that link these two. [7-8]

Population health vs. public health:
While related, population health and public health are distinct: [7-9]

Concept	Focus	Primary Actors	Key Methods	References
Public health	Health of the community as a whole; prevention of disease and promotion of health at the population level	Government agencies, public health departments	Surveillance, epidemiology, policy, regulation, health promotion	[1]
Population health	Health outcomes of a defined group AND the distribution of those outcomes; includes determinants	Healthcare systems, payers, communities, and public health	Data analytics, care management, social determinants interventions, cross-sector collaboration	[2-3]

Concept	Focus	Primary Actors	Key Methods	References
Population health management	Systematic approach to ensuring all members of a defined population receive appropriate care	Healthcare organizations, accountable care organizations	Registries, risk stratification, care coordination, quality improvement	[4]

[7-9][14]

Two uses of "population health" in academic medicine: [15]

1. **Clinical population health:** The health of a group of patients receiving care from a particular health system (e.g., "our diabetic population").
2. This is the focus of population health management, value-based care, and accountable care organizations.
3. **Community population health:** The health of people residing in a particular region or community, irrespective of where they receive care. This considers healthcare as one among many drivers of health status and maintains a focus on health equity.

Both perspectives are important for residents:

- **Clinical population health:** Managing your panel of continuity patients, ensuring they receive evidence-based preventive care, and identifying high-risk patients for initiative-taking outreach.
- **Community population health:** Understanding the social and environmental factors affecting your patients' health, partnering with community organizations, and advocating for policies that improve health.

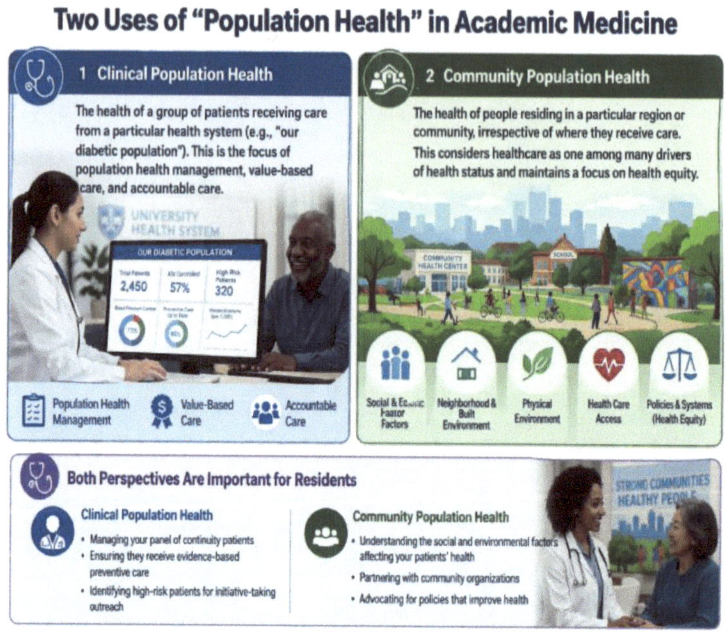

FIGURE *6.1 Two uses of population health in academic medicine.*

6.3 The 5As Framework for Social Determinants

The 5As framework provides a structured approach for clinicians to address biopsychosocial determinants in routine practice: Awareness, Adjustment, Assistance, Alignment, and Advocacy. Each represents a distinct level of engagement with the social context of a patient's care, from simple recognition through active policy advocacy.

Social and economic factors—such as those related to food, housing, and transportation—are major drivers of health and health inequities. Multiple national professional organizations have articulated roles for physicians in identifying and addressing social determinants of health (SDOH) and the need to include SDOH in all stages of physician education. [16-18]

The **5As framework** developed by the National Academies of Sciences, Engineering, and Medicine elaborates five strategies to strengthen social care: [16] [19-21]

1. Awareness – Identify social risks and assets through screening and assessment
What does this mean in practice:

- Screen patients for social needs using validated tools (e.g., PRAPARE, AHC-HRSN, WECARE)
- Ask about food security, housing stability, transportation, utilities, safety, and social support.
- Document social risks in the medical record.
- Recognize that social risks are clinical data, not just "social work issues."

Example: During your continuity clinic, you use a brief screening tool to identify that your patient with uncontrolled hypertension is experiencing food insecurity and cannot afford her medications.

2. Adjustment – Modify clinical care to account for social context
What does this mean in practice:

- Prescribe medications that patients can afford (use generic alternatives, $4 lists, patient assistance programs)
- Adjust treatment plans based on patients' living situations (e.g., insulin storage for homeless patients)
- Consider health literacy when providing education.
- Tailor follow-up frequency based on social support and access.

Example: Knowing your patient cannot afford her antihypertensive, you switch from a brand-name ARB to generic lisinopril and connect her with a patient assistance program.

3. Assistance – Provide direct support or navigation to community resources
What does this mean in practice:

- Connect patients to food banks, housing assistance, and transportation programs.

- Provide warm handoffs to social workers, community health workers, or patient navigators.
- Create and maintain resource directories for your clinic.
- Follow up to ensure patients access resources.

Example: You provide your patient with information about the local food bank and SNAP enrollment, and you place a referral to the clinic social worker for medication assistance.

4. Alignment – Coordinate care across health and social service sectors
What does this mean in practice:

- Build partnerships between your clinic/hospital and community organizations.
- Participating in community health needs assessments
- Engage in cross-sector collaborations (healthcare + housing, healthcare + education, etc.)
- Share data (with appropriate consent) across sectors to coordinate care.

Example: Your residency program partners with a local housing authority to provide on-site health services for residents of public housing, addressing both housing stability and healthcare access.

5. Advocacy – Work to change policies and systems that create health inequities

What does this mean in practice:

- Advocate for policies that address root causes of health inequities (e.g., minimum wage, housing policy, environmental justice)
- Participate in professional organizations that engage in policy advocacy.
- Educate policymakers about the health impacts of social policies.
- Support community organizing and civic engagement.

Example: You join your state medical association's advocacy committee and testify before the legislature about the health impacts of Medicaid expansion.

The following figure from Eder et al. published in JAMA illustrates the analytic framework for screening and interventions for social risk factors, showing the pathway from population screening through detection, intervention, and outcomes. [22]

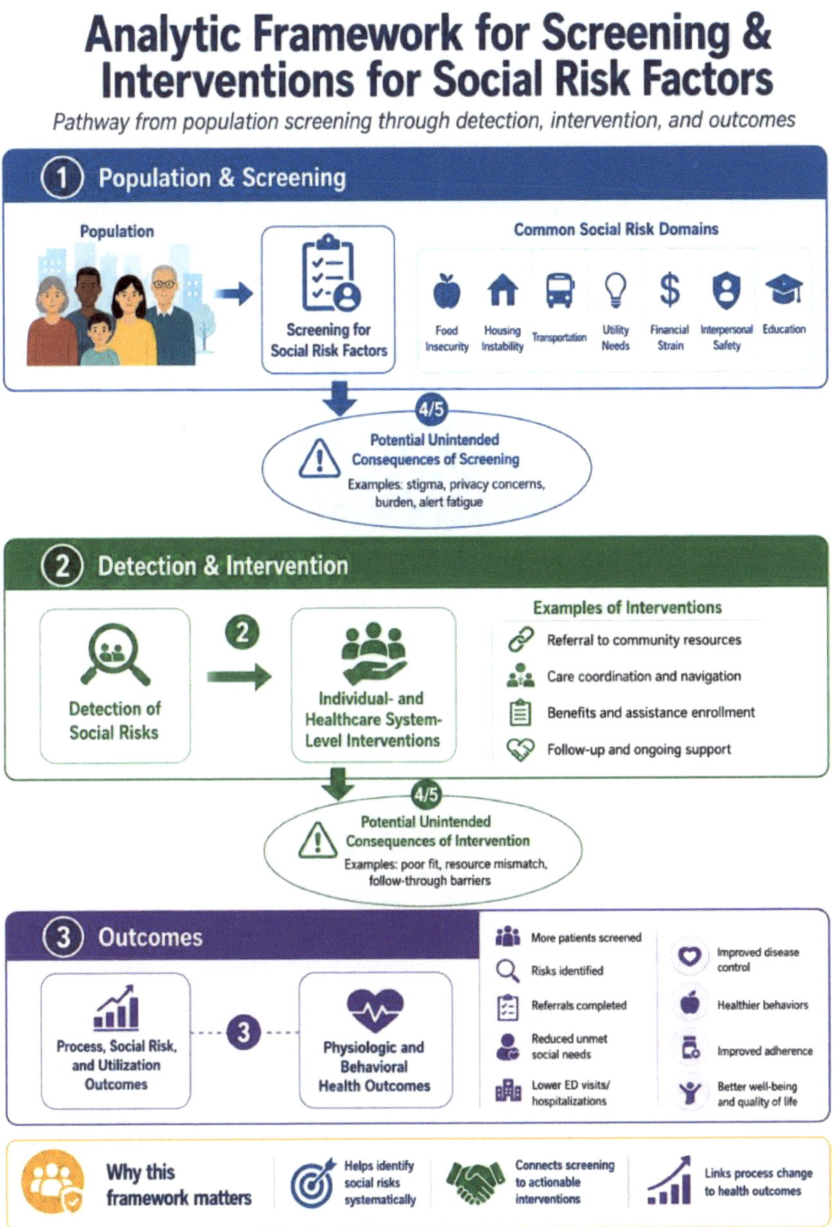

Adapted from Eder M, Henninger M, Durbin S, et al. Screening and Interventions for Social Risk Factors. JAMA. 2021.

6.4 Structural Racism and Health Inequities

Structural racism—the totality of ways in which societies foster racial discrimination through mutually reinforcing systems—is increasingly recognized as a fundamental cause of health inequity. It operates at three levels: institutional (policies and practices), interpersonal (individual interactions), and internalized (acceptance by stigmatized groups of negative messages).

The following figure from Amezcua et al. published in JAMA Neurology illustrates how structural racism leads to social determinants of health, which in turn produce health disparities and health inequities. [23]

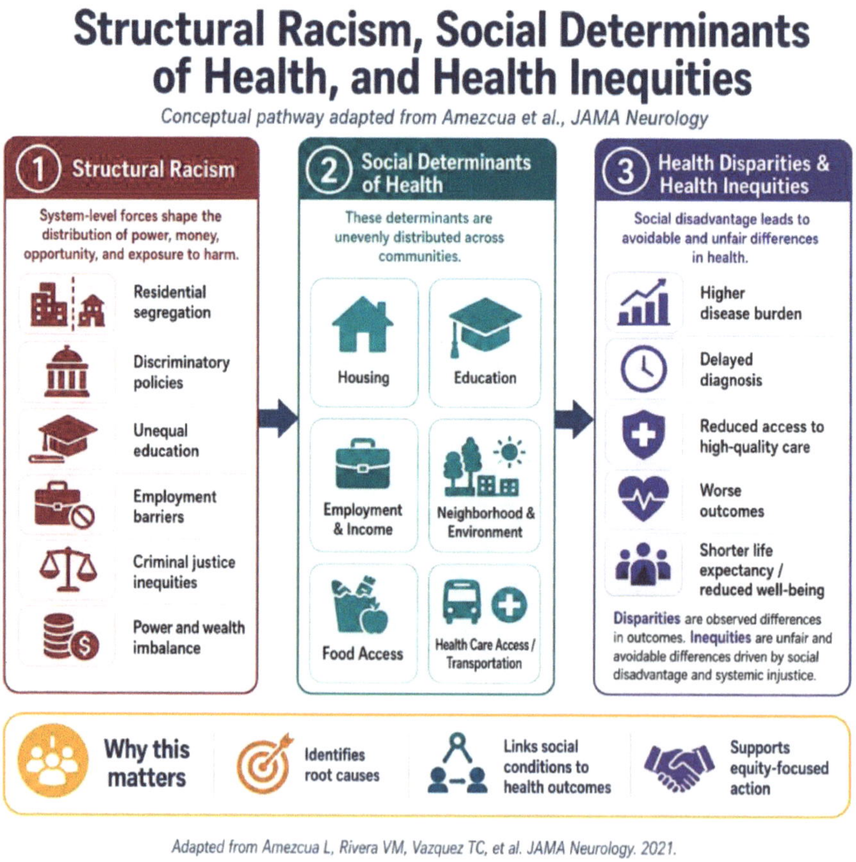

Key concepts:

Health disparities are negative differences in health linked to social, economic, and environmental disadvantages. [23]

Health inequities are shaped by differences in access to facilities and services linked to social disadvantages. [23]

Structural racism creates and maintains these disparities through:

- Prejudice, stereotype, and discrimination.
- Power and wealth imbalance
- Differential access to education, employment, housing, healthcare
- Environmental injustice
- Underrepresentation in research

Clinical implications:

- Recognize that disparities in outcomes (e.g., higher mortality from heart failure in Black patients) are not due to inherent biological differences, but to structural factors.
- Ensure your QI projects measure equity outcomes (reach and effectiveness by race, ethnicity, language, insurance status)
- Advocate for system-level interventions, not just individual-level solutions
- Engage community members as partners in designing and implementing interventions.

6.5 A Framework for Resident Participation

Several practical avenues exist for resident participation in population-health work: panel management, population-level QI, community partnership, public-health rotations, and advocacy/policy work.

A five-stage framework for residents' participation in population health initiatives has been proposed: [24]

Stage 1: Organize and Prepare

- Identify community partners and stakeholders.
- Understanding the community's health priorities and assets
- Build relationships with community organizations.
- Prepare residents with population health skills.

Stage 2: Plan and Prioritize

- Participating in community health needs assessments
- Use data to identify priority health issues.
- Engage community members in setting priorities.
- Align residency projects with community needs.

Stage 3: Implement

- Deploying evidence-based interventions
- Adapt interventions to local context.
- Engage in cross-sector collaboration.
- Document implementation processes.

Stage 4: Monitor and Evaluate

- Track process and outcome measures.
- Assess reach and equity.
- Identify barriers and facilitators.
- Use data for continuous improvement.

Stage 5: Sustain

- Build capacity within community organizations.
- Secure ongoing funding and resources
- Integrate successful interventions into routine practice.
- Hand off to community partners for long-term maintenance

Practical opportunities for residents: [24-27]

In continuity clinic:

- Manage your patient panel using registries and population health reports.
- Identify patients overdue for preventive care and conduct outreach.
- Screen for social determinants and connect patients to resources.
- Participate in clinic-based QI projects.

In the community:

- Participating in community health needs assessments
- Partner with community organizations on health promotion initiatives
- Conduct health education in schools, churches, or community centers.
- Engage in advocacy for policies that improve community health.

In the hospital:

- Improve transitions of care for high-risk patients.
- Address social needs during hospitalization (food, housing, transportation for discharge)
- Participate in readmission reduction initiatives.
- Engage in patient navigation and care coordination.

6.6 Civic Health and Medical Education

Civic health refers to the engagement of clinicians as citizens in the democratic processes that shape the social determinants of health. A growing body of work argues that civic health should be incorporated explicitly into medical education.

Why civic health matters for physicians: [28-29]

- **Health and civic engagement are reciprocally linked:** Healthier people participate more fully in civic life, and civically active people experience better health.
- **Social determinants of health are also drivers of civic engagement:** Poverty, racism, housing instability, and food insecurity reduce both health and civic participation.
- **Civic engagement is directly actionable:** Unlike many social determinants, civic engagement can be promoted through simple interventions.
- **Medical students and residents are effective messengers:** Patients trust healthcare providers, and providers can promote civic engagement during clinical encounters.

How to integrate civic health into your practice: [28]
Didactic opportunities:

- Attending lectures or panels on civic engagement and health
- Participate in discussions about the role of physicians in advocacy.
- Learn about the policy process and how to engage with policymakers.

Experiential opportunities:

- Distribute QR codes or information to aid in voter registration.
- Organize or participate in voter registration drives.
- Engage in nonpartisan canvassing or community organizing.
- Volunteer with community organizations addressing social determinants.

Clinical opportunities:

- Ask patients about barriers to civic participation (transportation, time, knowledge)
- Provide information about voter registration and civic resources.
- Connect patients to community organizations that promote civic engagement.

Because civic health is directly actionable, it can be a source of motivation rather than burnout for medical students and residents. As you develop as a medical professional, training in civic health deepens your understanding of social determinants and enables you to play a significant role in empowering patients with the democratic tools needed to enact social change. [28]

6.7 Integrating SDOH into Clinical Practice

Practical steps include adopting validated screening tools (PRAPARE, AHC HRSN); developing familiarity with the local resource landscape; documenting SDOH findings with ICD-10 Z codes; engaging social workers and case managers early; and tracking outcomes among patients with identified SDOH needs.

Step 1: Screen for social needs.

- Use a validated screening tool (PRAPARE, AHC-HRSN, WECARE, or your institution's tool)
- Integrate screening into routine clinical workflow (intake, annual visits, hospital admission)
- Document results in the medical record using ICD-10 Z codes.

Step 2: Adjust your clinical care.

- Consider social context when making treatment decisions.
- Prescribe affordable medications.
- Tailor education to health literacy level
- Adjust follow-up frequency based on social support and access.

Step 3: Help.

- Know your local resources (food banks, housing assistance, transportation, utility assistance)
- Create or use a community resource directory.
- Provide warm handoffs to social workers or community health workers.
- Follow up to ensure patients access resources.

Step 4: Advocate for alignment.

- Participating in community health needs assessments
- Support partnerships between your institution and community organizations.
- Engage in cross-sector collaborations.

Step 5: Engage in advocacy.

- Join professional organizations that advocate for health equity.
- Educate policymakers about the health impacts of social policies.
- Support community organizing and civic engagement.
- Vote and encourage your patients to vote.

6.8 The REVOLUTIONS Framework

The REVOLUTIONS framework is a recent proposal for the comprehensive incorporation of social accountability into medical education. The acronym identifies eleven constituent elements: Relevance, Equity, Voice, Outcomes, Long-term partnerships, Upstream focus, Transformative learning, Interprofessional collaboration, Operational integration, Networked institutions, and Sustainable funding.

From		Strategy		To
Individual focus MCAT examination score and grade point average	→	**Recruitment** Identify and cultivate potential students who are most likely to practice medicine as a socially accountable profession focused on community-identified needs[2]	→	**Global focus** Social action; pipeline programs
Clinical determinants Biological pathogenesis	→	**Environment** Embed issues of culture, context of care, history, and geographic place – all social determinants of health – in all curricular endeavors[3]	→	**Social determinants** Poverty, race, gender, and environment
Technical Disease-specific competencies	→	**Vocational development** Cultivate a sense of social contract through identity development recognizing how medical practice can address community-identified priority health concerns[4]	→	**Professional** Practice orientation: primary care and underserved settings
Patient centered Medical expert to individual patients	→	**Organizing systems** Promote a commitment to medical practice that serves societal needs, focused on marginalized populations and best attended to by interdisciplinary systems founded on principles of primary care[5]	→	**Community centered** Resource to a defined practice population
Prescription Biomedical treatment	→	**Leadership** Develop connection by expanding competencies from 1-on-1 patient-physician communication to community-based advocacy[6]	→	**Advocacy** Civic engagement
Knowledge Evidenced-based practice	→	**Understanding** Foster practical wisdom-based (needs-oriented) reasoning preferentially over rote learning of compartmentalized knowledge[7]	→	**Wisdom** Practice-based evidence
Traditional Conventional career oriented	→	**Training of faculty** Refocus faculty members toward participatory methods of education, research, and mentoring[8]	→	**Collaborative** Learner, community, and team oriented
Biomedical Bench research	→	**Investigation** Foster inquiry using community- and population-based methods[9]	→	**Participatory** COPC, CBPR, and QAOR
Disease model Hospital-based rotations	→	**Orientation** Support active and ongoing processes for identifying priority needs and developing action-oriented responses, using a systems model of iterative evaluation[10]	→	**Systems model** Longitudinal primary care clerkships
Medical competency Quality metrics	→	**Nurturance** Nurture physicians in socially accountable practices through suitable continuing education, leadership training, and appropriate incentives[11]	→	**Health citizenship** Community involvement
Individual obligation Accountable to single patient issues	→	**Social responsiveness** Enable teachers and learners proactively to address community needs, integrating public health with all levels of clinical medicine[12]	→	**Social need** Accountable to public priorities

REVOLUTIONS Framework for Socially Accountable Medical Education
Citizenship and Social Responsibility in Surgery: A Review. JAMA Surg. May 31, 2022.

Key transformations in the framework:

- From **individual focus** (MCAT scores, GPAs) to **global focus** (social action, pipeline programs)
- From **clinical determinants** (biological pathogenesis) to **social determinants** (poverty, environment)
- From **patient-centered** (care delivered by medical experts) to **community-centered** (care for defined practice populations)
- From **individual research** to **community-based participatory research**
- From **continuing medical education** to **continuing professional development** that includes advocacy and community engagement

Key Takeaways for Section 6:

✓ **The biopsychosocial model** provides a framework for understanding the complex, interacting factors that drive health and disease. Effective clinical care requires attention to biological, psychological, and social factors. [1] [3-4]

✓ **Population health** encompasses both clinical population health (managing your patient panel) and community population health (understanding and addressing the health of your community). [7-8][15]

✓ **The 5As framework** (Awareness, Adjustment, Assistance, Alignment, Advocacy) provides a practical structure for addressing social determinants of health in clinical practice. [16][19]

✓ **Structural racism** is a root cause of health disparities and inequities. Implementation science for equity must address structural factors, not just individual behaviors. [23]

✓ **Residents can participate in population health** through panel management, community partnerships, QI projects, and advocacy. [24-26]

✓ **Civic health** is directly actionable and can be promoted through simple interventions in clinical settings. Medical students and residents are effective messengers of civic engagement. [28-29]

✓ **Socially accountable medical education** requires transformation across all dimensions of training, from recruitment to continuing professional development. [30]

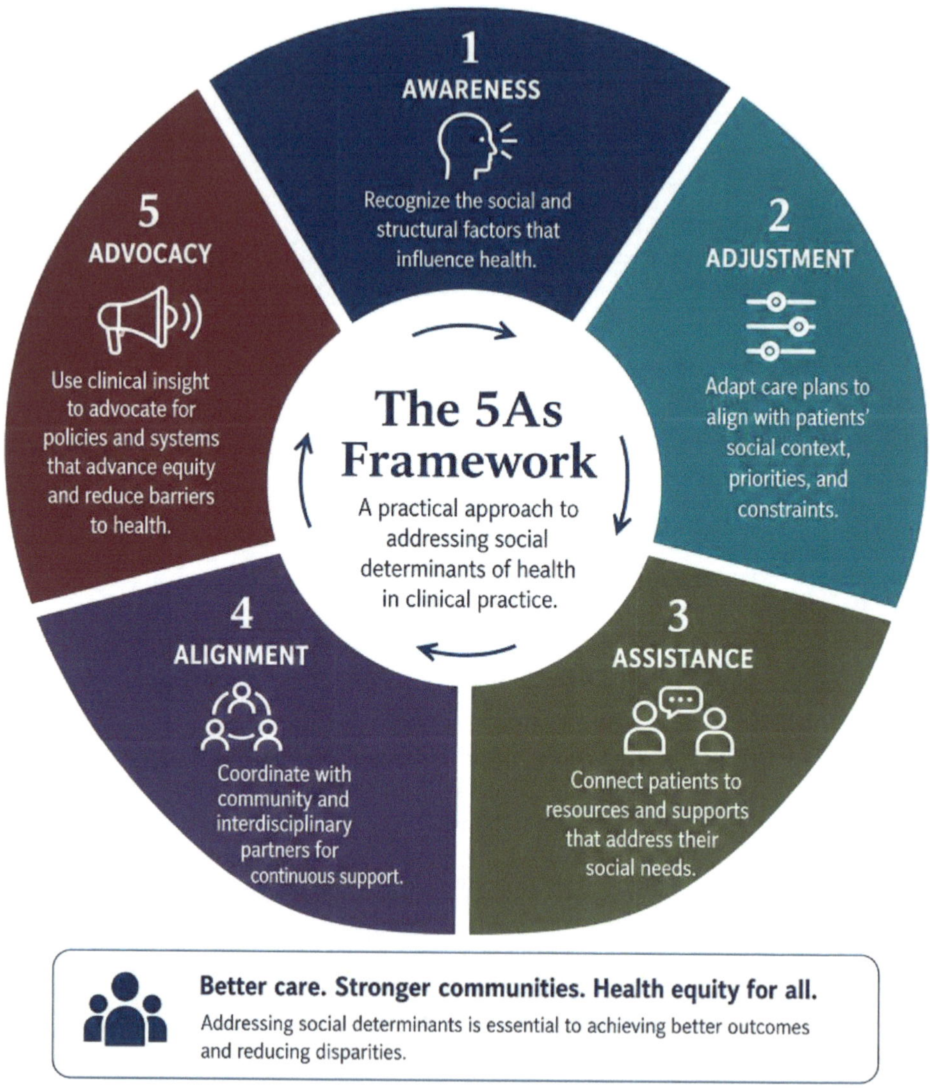
The 5As Framework
A practical approach to addressing social determinants of health in clinical practice.
1
AWARENESS
Recognize the social and structural factors that influence health.
2
ADJUSTMENT
Adapt care plans to align with patients' social context, priorities, and constraints.
3
ASSISTANCE
Connect patients to resources and supports that address their social needs.
4
ALIGNMENT
Coordinate with community and interdisciplinary partners for continuous support.
5
ADVOCACY
Use clinical insight to advocate for policies and systems that advance equity and reduce barriers to health.
Better care. Stronger communities. Health equity for all.
Addressing social determinants is essential to achieving better outcomes and reducing disparities.

CHAPTER 7

Digital Health and AI Competencies

7.1 The DECODE Framework

The **Digital Health Competencies in Medical Education (DECODE) framework**, developed through an international Delphi consensus process, articulates a shared, future-oriented vision of what medical graduates should be able to do in an increasingly digital health ecosystem. Rather than treating digital health as an optional add-on or a technical niche, the DECODE framework positions it as a core component of professional identity and day-one readiness for practice. It specifies a set of digital-health competencies that are expected of all new physicians, organized across **six principal domains**: **data literacy, evidence appraisal, communication, operational use, design and improvement, and ethics**.

Data literacy encompasses the ability to understand, interpret, and critically use health data—from electronic health records and registries to patient-generated data and digital biomarkers.

Evidence appraisal focuses on evaluating digital tools and interventions (such as apps, AI decision support, and remote monitoring platforms) using rigorous clinical and methodological standards.

Communication addresses how clinicians interact with patients, families, and colleagues through digital channels, including telemedicine, patient portals, and asynchronous messaging, while maintaining clarity, empathy, and professionalism.

Operational use involves the practical skills required to navigate digital systems safely and efficiently in real clinical workflows, including documentation, order entry, and information retrieval.

Design and improvement highlight the role of clinicians as co-designers and improvers of digital tools and systems, contributing frontline insight to user-centered design, usability testing, and iterative refinement.

Finally, **ethics** emphasizes responsible, equitable, and transparent use of digital technologies, including attention to privacy, bias, accountability, and impact of digital systems on patient autonomy and trust.

The DECODE framework comprises four domains:

Table 2. Description of Domains

Domain	Importance	Description
Professionalism in digital health	The use of digital technologies in health care poses important professional, legal, and ethical implications, and demands a high level of medical professionalism.	This domain encompasses themes that are related to professionalism in digital health, which is described as the ability of health professionals to understand, develop, and demonstrate appropriate professional behavior when using digital technologies. Learning outcomes within this domain prepare medical graduates to become competent and responsible digital health users with an awareness of cybersecurity and ethical, legal, and regulatory guidelines and demonstrate digital intelligence. Mastery of this domain will allow them to incorporate technologies in their daily practice without compromising data of their patients.
Patient and population digital health	A widespread availability of internet, mobile, and wearable technologies empowers patients and healthy individuals to be active participants (ie, digital health consumers) in the process of making choices about their health, rather than being recipients of services. This trend allows for person-centered care; the prerequisites for that include a focus on patient in informatics, promotion of digital health literacy, and patient education.	This domain focuses on equipping medical students with knowledge and skills in telehealth, health apps, digital therapeutics, wearables, sensors, remote monitoring, and point-of-care and self-testing. It enables them to communicate, counsel, provide care, and motivate self-management in patients in the context of digital health technologies. It also expands on the types of data that can be collected through digital technologies available to patients and how this may lead to better diagnoses and treatment decisions in the future. Additionally, it ensures medical students are aware of digital health literacy of patients, the broader digital determinants of health, the digital divide, and associated health inequalities.
Health information systems	Physicians, among other health care professionals, are key stakeholders in collecting, storing, monitoring, accessing, and sharing patient health data. Accurate and safe handling of health data extends beyond the quality and safety requirement of an individual patient's care. Clinical decision support systems, computerized physician order entries, and other information technology solutions embedded within health information systems leverage existing health data and enhance patient care by providing automation and decision support.	Competencies in this domain prepare medical students to be competent users of health information systems and health information exchange who are aware of the design and development process of such systems. It ensures that medical students are compliant with the standards of data governance policies. Furthermore, it focuses on clinical documentation skills and electronic prescribing methods.
Health data science	The growth of digitally captured, processed, and stored health data has been drastic, creating opportunities to address challenges in medicine, public health, and biomedical sciences. In addition to data from electronic health records, patient-generated data (eg, wearables) and genome sequencing contribute substantially to the health data pool. One of the promises of this trend is the use of multiple modalities to support personalized medicine.	This domain covers competencies in health data application fields such as population health informatics, computational thinking, artificial intelligence in health care, and precision medicine. It ensures medical students understand the scope of health data, the impact of data on health care, and how to apply data for the optimization of patient care at both the population and individual levels.

Description of Domains
The Digital Health Competencies in Medical Education Framework: An International Consensus Statement Based on a Delphi Study. JAMA New Open. January 1, 2025.

Domain 1: Professionalism in Digital Health

This domain encompasses appropriate professional behavior when using digital technologies, including:

- **Digital professionalism:** Maintaining professional boundaries on social media, protecting patient privacy in digital communications, and understanding the permanence of digital footprints.
- **Cybersecurity:** Recognizing phishing attempts, using secure passwords, protecting patient data from breaches
- **Ethical, legal, and regulatory considerations:** Understanding HIPAA, informed consent for digital health tools, and liability.
- **Digital intelligence:** Critical evaluation of online health information, recognizing misinformation.

Clinical application: When you post on social media, even on personal accounts, you represent the medical profession. Never post identifiable patient information, avoid disparaging comments about patients or colleagues, and be aware that your online presence affects patient trust.

Domain 2: Patient and Population Digital Health

This domain focuses on patient-facing digital technologies:

- **Digital health literacy:** Recognizing that patients have varying abilities to access, understand, and use digital health information; addressing the digital divide.
- **Telehealth:** Conducting effective video and phone visits, recognizing limitations, ensuring appropriate use
- **Digital diagnostics:** Using AI-assisted diagnostic tools, point-of-care testing, and remote monitoring.
- **Wearables and sensors:** Interpreting data from fitness trackers, continuous glucose monitors, smartwatches
- **Health apps and digital therapeutics:** Recommending evidence-based apps, understanding FDA-cleared digital therapeutics.
- **Digital determinants of health:** Recognizing how the lack of internet access, digital literacy, or devices creates health inequities.

Clinical application: Before recommending a patient portal or health app, assess the patient's digital literacy, internet access, and device availability. A patient without a smartphone or reliable internet cannot benefit from a patient portal—and may feel excluded if you assume they can.

Domain 3: Health Information Systems

This domain prepares you to be a competent user of health information technology:

- **Data governance and management:** Understanding how health data is collected, stored, and protected.
- **Electronic health records (EHRs):** Efficient documentation, electronic prescribing, using clinical decision support, avoiding alert fatigue.
- **Health information exchange:** Understanding how data flows between systems, and interoperability challenges.
- **Human-centered design:** Evaluating whether digital tools are designed with users (clinicians and patients) in mind.

Clinical application: EHR documentation is a major source of physician burnout. Learn efficient documentation strategies: use templates appropriately, leverage voice recognition, avoid copy-paste errors, and document for communication (not just billing).

Domain 4: Health Data Science

This domain covers analytical and computational aspects of digital health:

- **Public health informatics:** Using data for population health surveillance, outbreak detection, and quality reporting.
- **Artificial intelligence in healthcare:** Understanding AI/ML concepts, evaluating AI tools, recognizing limitations and biases.
- **Computational thinking:** Applying logical, algorithmic thinking to clinical problems.
- **Precision medicine:** Understanding how genomic and other data enable personalized treatment.

Clinical application: When your hospital implements a new AI-based sepsis alert, you should be able to ask: What data does it use? How was it validated? What is the false positive rate? Does it perform equally well across patient populations?

7.2 Artificial Intelligence in Clinical Practice

Artificial intelligence in clinical practice ranges from established techniques in medical imaging interpretation through clinical-decision-support tools, ambient documentation assistants, and predictive analytics, to emerging applications of large language models in clinical communication and synthesis.

Types of AI in healthcare: [2]

- **Machine learning:** Computational techniques that learn from examples instead of operating from predefined rules (e.g., risk prediction models, image classification)
- **Natural language processing (NLP):** The ability of a computer to transform human language and unstructured text into machine-readable structured data (e.g., extracting diagnoses from clinical notes, ambient scribes)
- **Generative AI:** AI that can create updated content, including text, images, and code (e.g., ChatGPT, clinical documentation assistants)

Current high-value uses of AI: [2-4]

- **Medical imaging:** Diabetic retinopathy screening, mammography interpretation, chest X-ray analysis, pathology slide review
- **Clinical decision support:** Sepsis prediction, deterioration alerts, drug interaction checking, diagnostic suggestions.
- **Administrative tasks:** Scheduling optimization, prior authorization, revenue cycle management, clinical documentation
- **Patient engagement:** Chatbots for triage, medication reminders, symptom checkers

The application-readiness cadence:
Different AI applications are at distinct stages of maturity and carry distinct levels of risk. The following figure from Maddox et al. published in NEJM illustrates how AI applications should be deployed based on their risk-opportunity profile, with lower-risk applications (like patient education) ready for near-term deployment while higher-risk applications (like treatment decision support) require longer development timelines and more rigorous validation. [5]

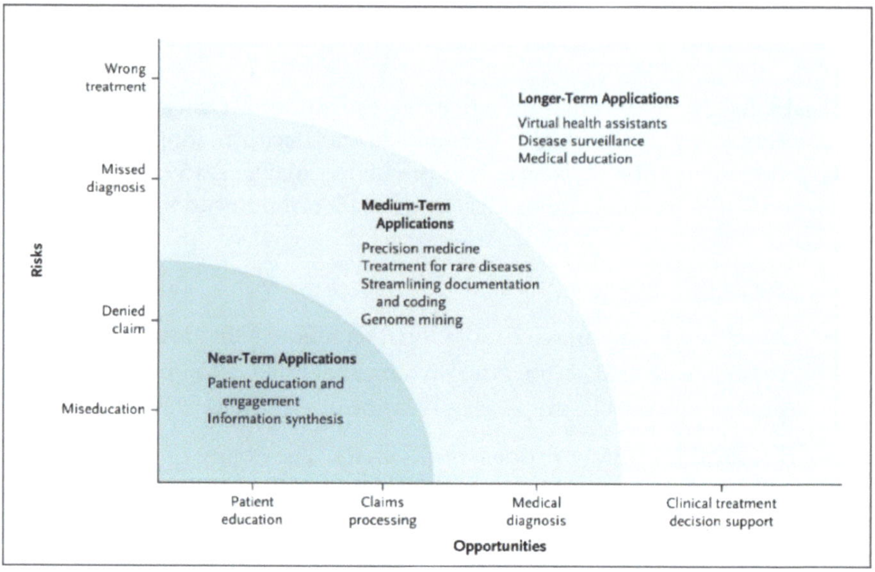

Application-Readiness Cadence for Large Language Models. Generative AI in Medicine — Evaluating Progress and Challenges. N Engl J Med. June 25, 2025.

7.3 Critical Appraisal of AI Tools

Every clinician should be able to ask, and to seek answers to, a structured set of questions before adopting an AI tool in clinical practice.

APPRAISAL QUESTIONS FOR AN AI TOOL

Validation: On what population was the model trained by? Has it been validated in external datasets? What are its performance characteristics in the deployment population?

Bias & equity: Has it been tested for differential performance across demographic groups?

Workflow integration: Does it generate alert fatigue, or is it surfaced only when actionable?

Outcome impact: Has its use been shown to improve outcomes? What is the risk of automation bias?

Governance: Is the model regulated as a medical device? Who monitors ongoing performance after deployment?

Not all AI tools are created equal. Most uses of AI in healthcare delivery have not been subject to randomized controlled trials, and the usual level of evidence required for medical decision-making may be lacking. [2] As a clinician, you need to critically evaluate AI tools before trusting their outputs.

Key questions to ask about any AI tool: [6-9]

1. What problem is this tool trying to solve?

- Is this a real clinical problem that matters to patients?
- Is AI the right solution, or would a simpler approach work?
- Does the tool address a genuine need, or is it a solution looking for a problem?

2. How was the tool developed and validated?

- What data was used to train the model? (Size, source, representativeness)
- Was it validated on an independent dataset?
- Was it evaluated in a setting similar to yours?
- Were there randomized controlled trials, or only retrospective studies?

3. How does the tool perform?

- What is the sensitivity and specificity?
- What is the positive predictive value in your population?
- What is the false positive rate? (Alert fatigue is a real problem)
- How does performance compare to clinician judgment alone?

4. Is the tool fair and unbiased?

- Was performance evaluated across demographic groups (race, ethnicity, age, sex, socioeconomic status)?
- Are there known biases in the training data?
- Could the tool worsen health disparities?

5. Is the tool explainable and interpretable?

- Can you understand why the tool made a particular recommendation?
- Can you explain it to patients?
- Is there a "black box" problem?

6. How does the tool integrate into clinical workflow?

- Does it fit into existing workflows, or does it create extra work?
- Who is responsible for acting on the tool's output?
- What happens when the tool is wrong?

7. What are the governance and accountability structures?

- Who is responsible if the tool causes harm?
- How is the tool monitored for performance drift?
- Is there a process for reporting adverse events?

8. What are the costs and resource requirements?

- What does the tool cost (licensing, implementation, maintenance)?
- What training is required?
- Is the return on investment justified?

7.4 Human Values in AI

The design and deployment of AI tools embed value choices about what is to be optimized. The choice to train a clinical predictor on historical data expresses a judgment that the historical pattern of care is appropriate for future care judgment that becomes fraught when the historical pattern reflects systemic disparity. Clinicians are properly involved in these value choices.

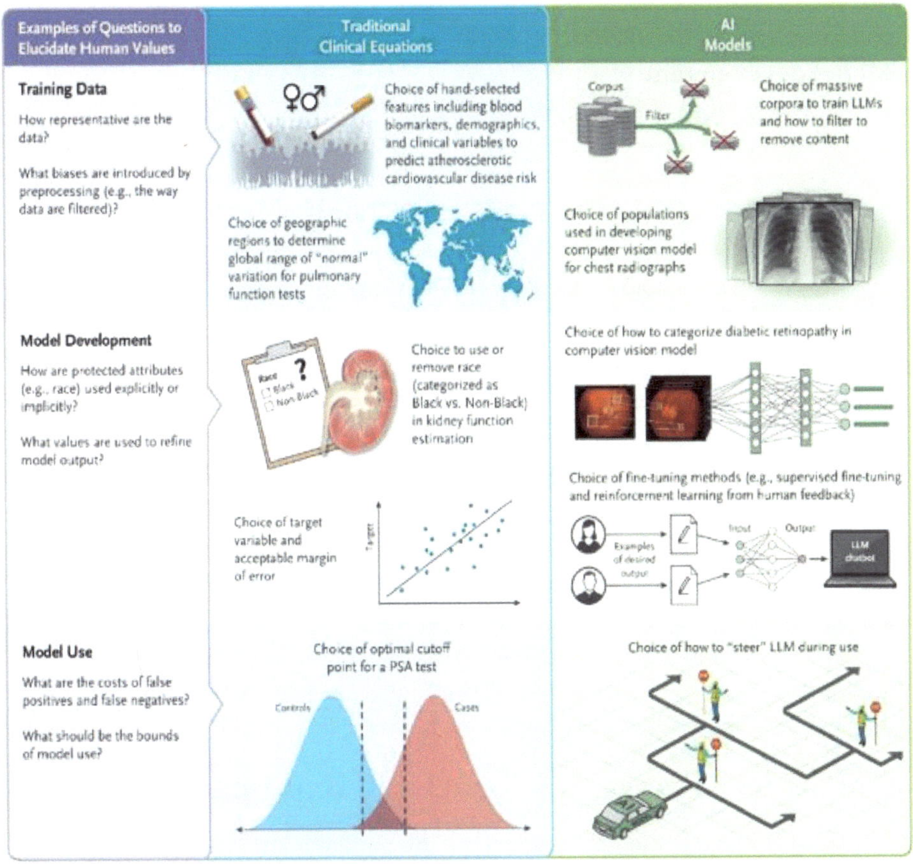

Entry Points and Choices for Human Values in Traditional Clinical Equations and New Artificial Intelligence Models.
Medical Artificial Intelligence and Human Values. N Engl J Med. May 29, 2024.

Key value-laden decisions in AI development:

Training data:

- Whose data is included? (If training data underrepresents certain populations, the model may perform poorly for those groups)
- What outcomes are measured? (If the outcome is "healthcare costs" rather than "health outcomes," the model may perpetuate existing inequities)
- How are missing data managed?

Model development:

- What features are included? (Should race be a variable? What about socioeconomic proxies?)
- How are errors weighed? (Is a false negative worse than a false positive?)
- What threshold is used for predictions?

Model use:

- Who has access to the tool?
- How are outputs communicated to clinicians and patients?
- What actions are triggered by the tool's recommendations?

Clinical implication: When you use an AI tool, you are implicitly accepting the value judgments embedded in its design. Be aware of these choices and their implications for your patients.

7.5 Ethical Principles for AI in Healthcare

- **Beneficence** – the tool must serve the patient's interest.
- **Non-maleficence** – the tool must not cause harm, particularly at scale.
- **Autonomy** – patients should be informed of AI's role in their care.
- **Justice** – benefits and burdens should be distributed equitably.

- **Transparency** – operation should be sufficiently understandable to support oversight.
- **Accountability** – clear responsibility for AI-assisted decisions.

Principles derived from medical ethics:

- **Beneficence:** AI should aim to do good and improve patient outcomes
- **Nonmaleficence:** AI should not cause harm; "safe failure" should be designed in
- **Autonomy:** Patients should have the right to know when AI is used in their care and to opt out
- **Justice:** AI should be fair and should not worsen health disparities

Principles derived from AI engineering:

- **Explainability:** The technology should be explainable in plain terms.
- **Interpretability:** There should be plausible reasoning for decisions
- **Fairness:** AI should be free from bias
- **Dependability:** AI should be dependable and fail safely
- **Audit trail:** Decisions should be traceable and reviewable.
- **Active management:** Knowledge base should be kept up to date.

Organizational principles:

- **Benevolence:** Organizations should aim to do good through AI
- **Transparency:** All assumptions and conflicts of interest should be declared
- **Accountability:** There should be active oversight and risk management

Special attention to vulnerable populations: Extreme care must be exercised when AI is used with vulnerable populations, including children, elderly, cognitively impaired, and socioeconomically disadvantaged individuals. [6]

7.6 Challenges to AI Implementation

Recurring challenges include distribution shift, alert fatigue, workflow disruption, equity concerns, liability ambiguity, and regulatory evolution. Each requires explicit attention during deployment planning rather than discovery as a post-implementation problem.

Despite the promise of AI, implementation faces significant challenges. The following figure from Sahni and Carrus, published in NEJM, illustrates the key barriers to AI adoption in healthcare delivery organizations. [2]

	Categories of Successful AI Deployment	Goal	Challenges
Strategic Vision	1 Mission-led road map	Ensure a clear view of where the value is going to be and a road map to get there	**Part of the Solution:** Ongoing belief that AI is a "silver bullet" rather than part of a broader solution **Transformative Potential:** Focusing only on the "incremental" opportunity rather than reimagining for the "transformative" potential **Total Mission Value:** Focusing only on financial factors rather than accounting for nonfinancial factors such as quality improvement, patient safety, patient experience, clinician satisfaction, and increased access to care **Focus:** Pursuing many domains rather than 1 or 2 "priority" domains with multiple uses of AI **Timing to Impact:** Misconception that AI is a "quick win" rather than a process that is implemented over multiple years
Key Enabling Factors	2 Talent	Ensure that the correct skills and capabilities are available to execute and innovate	**Skills:** Missing skill sets in workforce to implement and manage AI **Talent Road Map:** Lack of long-term plan for workforce hiring, upskilling, and reskilling as AI use expands **Education:** Underinvestment in making workforce AI-literate
	3 Agile delivery	Increase the speed at which teams are able to deliver work	**Culture:** Negative attitude toward AI or lack of consensus **Funding:** Limited ongoing funding to deploy AI
	4 Technology and tooling	Allow the organization to move quickly, with flexibility and resiliency	**Technology Infrastructure:** Inability to integrate AI into legacy systems, secure AI, or provide necessary computing power **Data Preparation:** Underinvestment in tools to properly prepare data
	5 Data management	Use data intelligence to derive a competitive advantage	**Completeness:** Inability to address data gaps with the use of internal or external sources **Unbiased Data:** Lack of awareness of inherent biases in data, such as data that are limited to one health system site **Availability:** Missing scale in the number of data points to train AI **Data Governance:** Governance to manage data is not formalized
Implementation	6 Change in operating model of the organization	Develop business processes, employee skills, and structures to realize total mission value	**Change Management:** Lack of recognition that translating strategic vision requires different behavior changes for everyone in the workforce, as well as coaching **Workflow Integration:** Failure to integrate AI into clinical workflow to minimize the behavior change needed **Cross-functional Teams:** Not creating fully cross-functional teams, such as clinicians, technologists, and operations professionals **Transparency:** Inability to overcome "black box" nature of AI, such as quantification of assumptions **Interpretable Output:** Not providing easy-to-understand output with relevant information to enhance decision making **Operational Governance:** Not creating a formal governance structure to oversee all aspects of implementation and ongoing management

Examples of Challenges to AI Adoption in Health Care Delivery Organizations.
Artificial Intelligence in the U.S. Health Care Delivery. N Engl J Med. July 26, 2023.

Key challenges: [2][9][11]

Strategic challenges:

- **Misunderstanding AI deployment:** Organizations often treat AI as a quick fix rather than a multi-year transformation process.
- **Narrow focus on financial returns:** Ignoring quality and safety benefits.
- **Lack of clear use cases:** Implementing AI without a clear problem to solve

Talent challenges:

- **Shortage of AI expertise:** Few healthcare organizations have data scientists, ML engineers, or clinical informaticists.
- **Lack of clinician AI literacy:** Clinicians do not know how to evaluate or use AI tools.
- **Change Resistance:** Clinicians may distrust AI or fear job displacement.

Technical challenges:

- **Data quality and interoperability:** Healthcare data is often fragmented, incomplete, or inconsistent.
- **EHR Integration:** AI tools must fit into existing workflows.
- **Model drift:** AI performance may degrade over time as patient populations or clinical practices change.

Governance challenges:

- **Regulatory uncertainty:** FDA oversight of AI is evolving; many tools are not regulated.
- **Liability concerns:** Who is responsible when AI causes harm?
- **Privacy concerns:** AI requires large datasets, raising privacy issues.

Equity challenges:

- **Algorithmic bias:** AI trained on biased data may perpetuate worsen disparities.
- **Digital divide:** AI may benefit patients with digital access while leaving others behind
- **Lack of diverse representation:** AI development teams often lack diversity.

7.7 Telemedicine Competencies

Telemedicine, formerly marginal, is now central to contemporary practice. Competence includes appropriateness assessment, webwide manners, troubleshooting technology, documentation and billing, and attention to equity—since telemedicine can widen disparities where patients lack broadband or digital literacy.

Core telemedicine competencies: [1][13]

Communication skills:

- Establishing rapport through a screen
- Using verbal and nonverbal cues effectively
- Managing technical difficulties gracefully
- Ensuring patient understanding through teach-back.

Data gathering:

- Conducting a focused history via video or phone
- Guiding patients through self-examination
- Knowing when physical examination is essential and telemedicine is inappropriate.
- Using peripheral devices (digital stethoscopes, otoscopes) when available

Clinical decision-making:

- Recognizing which conditions are appropriate for telemedicine.
- Knowing when to escalate to in-person care
- Documenting telemedicine encounters appropriately
- Managing prescribing in telemedicine (controlled substances, new medications)

Patient safety:

- Verifying patient identity and location
- Ensuring privacy on both ends
- Having a plan for emergencies during telemedicine visits
- Recognizing signs of abuse or coercion

Equity considerations:

- Assessing patients' access to technology and internet
- Offering audio-only options when video is not feasible.
- Providing interpreter services for telemedicine
- Avoiding assumptions about who can or cannot use telemedicine.

When telemedicine is appropriate: [12][14]

- **Chronic disease management:** Follow-up visits for stable conditions (diabetes, hypertension, heart failure)
- **Mental health:** Psychotherapy, medication management, crisis intervention
- **Post-operative follow-up:** Wound checks, symptom assessment
- **Medication management:** Refills, dose adjustments, side effect monitoring
- **Patient education:** Disease education, lifestyle counseling
- **Triage:** Determining need for in-person evaluation

When telemedicine is NOT appropriate: [12][14]

- **Acute emergencies:** Chest pain, stroke symptoms, severe dyspnea
- **Conditions requiring physical examination:** New abdominal pain, new neurological symptoms, skin lesions requiring palpation.
- **Procedures:** Any intervention requiring firsthand care
- **Patients who prefer in-person care:** Respect patient preferences
- **Situations where privacy cannot be ensured:** Patient in public places, concerns about coercion.

7.8 Practical Skills with the EHR

Effective use of the electronic health record is itself a clinical competency: efficient navigation, structured documentation, order-set use, decisions **EHR use is a major source of physician burnout**, with physicians spending two hours on EHR tasks for every hour of direct patient care. Efficient EHR skills early in your training will serve you throughout your career. [15]

EHR competencies for residents: [1][15]

Documentation:

- Use templates appropriately (but customize for each patient)
- Avoid copy-paste errors (review and update all copied text)
- Document for communication, not just billing
- Use structured data when possible (problem lists, medication lists)
- Learn voice recognition if available.

Order entry:

- Use order sets appropriately (but review each order)
- Understand clinical decision support alerts (do not just click through)
- Know how to find and use evidence-based order sets.
- Understand the difference between routine, urgent, and STAT orders.

Information retrieval:

- Navigate efficiently to find relevant information.
- Use search functions effectively.
- Know how to access outside records.
- Understand how to use clinical decision support tools.

Population health:

- Use patient registries to identify care gaps.
- Generate reports on your patient panel.
- Use EHR data for quality improvement.

Communication:

- Use secure messaging appropriately.
- Manage inboxes efficiently.
- Coordinate care through the EHR.

Privacy and security:

- Log out when leaving workstations.
- Never share passwords.
- Report on suspected breaches
- Understand audit trails.
- Support engagement, and data export for QI work.

7.9 The DATA-MD Curriculum: AI Literacy for Residents

The **Data-Augmented, Technology-Assisted Medical Decision Making (DATA-MD) curriculum** provides a model for teaching AI and machine learning concepts to clinical trainees. [16] The curriculum contains four modules:

Module 1: Introduction to AI/ML in Healthcare

- Definitions of AI, machine learning, deep learning
- Types of AI applications in healthcare
- Current state of AI adoption

Module 2: Epidemiology and Biostatistics in AI/ML

- Training, validation, and test sets
- Overfitting and underfitting
- Performance metrics (sensitivity, specificity, AUC, calibration)
- Bias and confounding in AI.

Module 3: Use of AI/ML to Augment Diagnostic Decisions

- AI in medical imaging
- Clinical decision support systems
- Risk prediction models.
- Integrating AI into clinical workflow

Module 4: Ethical and Legal Considerations of AI/ML in Healthcare

- Algorithmic bias and fairness
- Explainability and transparency
- Privacy and data security
- Liability and accountability
- Informed consent for AI

Outcomes: In the pilot study, learners showed significant improvements in knowledge scores for modules 1-3 and reported increased confidence in their abilities to appraise AI literature and use AI tools in future practice. [16]

7.10 Developing Your Digital Health Skills: Practical Steps

During medical school:

- Complete online modules on digital health (IHI Open School, Coursera, edX)
- Participate in telemedicine experiences during clinical rotations.
- Learn to use the EHR efficiently during clerkships.
- Take electives in clinical informatics if available.
- Attend grand rounds or seminars on AI in healthcare.

During residency:

- Seeking out telemedicine clinic experiences
- Participating in EHR optimization committees

- Lead or participate in QI projects involving health IT.
- Critically evaluate AI tools used in your institution.
- Consider clinical informatics elective or rotation.

Resources for learning:

Resource	What It Offers	Access
IHI Open School	Free courses on QI, patient safety, and health IT	ihi.org/education
AMIA 10x10 Program	Introduction to clinical informatics	amia.org
Coursera/edX	AI and machine learning courses	coursera.org, edx.org
AAMC Telehealth Competencies	Framework for telehealth education	aamc.org
FDA Digital Health Center	Information on regulated digital health tools	fda.gov/medical-devices/digital-health
AMA Digital Health Playbook	Practical guidance for physicians	ama-assn.org

[1][13] [16-17]

Key Takeaways for Section 7:

✓ **Digital health competencies are essential** for modern medical practice. The DECODE framework provides a comprehensive roadmap across four domains: professionalism, patient/population health, health information systems, and health data science. [1]

✓ **AI is already in your clinical environment.** Learn to critically evaluate AI tools by asking about their development, validation, performance, fairness, explainability, and integration into workflow. [2] [6-7]

✓ **AI tools embed human values** at every stage of development. Be aware of the choices made in data selection, model design, and implementation, and their implications for your patients. [10]

✓ **Telemedicine is here to stay.** Develop competencies in communication, data gathering, clinical decision-making, and patient safety for virtual visits. [12-13]

✓ **EHR efficiency is a career-long skill.** Learn to document effectively, use clinical decision support appropriately, and leverage EHR data for population health. [15]

✓ **Equity must be central** to digital health implementation. Recognize the digital divide, algorithmic bias, and the potential for technology to worsen disparities if not implemented thoughtfully. [1][8][12]

✓ **Continuous learning is essential.** Digital health is evolving rapidly; commit to ongoing education throughout your career. [16-17]

CHAPTER 8

Health Parity in Implementation Science

Health equity is not an optional add-on to implementation science—it is foundational. As Brownson and colleagues argue, **"Every project in implementation science should include a parity focus."** For some studies, equity is the central goal; for others, it is one consideration among many. [1] But at minimum, every implementation effort should ensure that existing disparities are not widened and that no population is left behind.

As a senior medical student or resident, you will care for patients from diverse backgrounds, many of whom experience health inequities rooted in structural factors beyond their individual control. Understanding how to design, implement, and evaluate interventions through an equity lens is essential for your development as a physician-leader.

8.1 Defining Health Parity and Health Disparities

Health disparities are negative differences in health linked to social, economic, and environmental disadvantages. [2] These are the measurable differences in health outcomes between groups.

Health disproportions are shaped by differences in access to facilities and services linked to social disadvantages. [2] These are the unfair and avoidable differences that result from systemic factors.

Health parity shifts focus from shortcomings to attainable goals, promoting a positive outlook on societal progress. [1] Health equity means that everyone has a fair and just opportunity to be as healthy as possible.

Why the distinction matters:

- **Disparities** describe the problem (e.g., Black patients with heart failure have higher mortality than White patients)
- **Disproportions** identify the cause (e.g., structural racism, differential access to care, implicit bias)
- **Parity** defines the goal (e.g., all patients with heart failure receive guideline-directed medical therapy regardless of race)

Implementation of science and parity:
Implementation science has the potential to reduce disparities by understanding factors such as structural racism, socioeconomic deprivation, social bias, and innate healthcare system barriers that create disparities. Implementation scientists can develop interventions and strategies to reduce inequities, including developing antiracism interventions, training healthcare professionals to deliver culturally sensitive care, or implementing policy changes to improve access to care for disenfranchised communities. [3]

However, **implementation of science can also worsen disparities** if not designed with equity in mind. QI interventions aimed at improving overall quality may not reduce disparities and, in some cases, may worsen them if the intervention is adopted more widely or is more effective among the population with better baseline outcomes. [4]

8.2 Why Do QI Projects Can Worsen Disparities

The "rising tide" problem:
A common assumption in quality improvement is that "a rising tide lifts all boats"—that improving overall quality will benefit everyone equally. This is often false. QI projects designed without an intentional focus on equity promotion may foster **intervention-generated inequalities** that further disadvantage vulnerable groups. [5]

How this happens:
Differential reach: An intervention may be more accessible to patients with resources (transportation, time off work, internet access, health literacy)

Differential effectiveness: An intervention may work better for patients who are already healthier, more engaged, or have more social support.

Differential adoption: Providers may be more likely to offer interventions to patients they perceive as "compliant" or "motivated."

Differential sustainability: Improvements may be sustained in well-resourced settings but fade in under-resourced settings.

Example: A hospital implements a patient portal to improve medication adherence. Overall adherence improves by 15%.
But when stratified by race:

- White patients: 20% improvement
- Black patients: 8% improvement
- Hispanic patients: 5% improvement

The intervention widened the disparity because it was more accessible and effective for patients with internet access, digital literacy, and English proficiency.

The solution: **Parity-focused quality improvement (EF-QI)**
EF-QI differs from QI with an equity lens in that it is action-oriented and centered around equity. EF-QI initiatives purposely integrate equity throughout the fabric of the project and are inclusive, collaborative efforts that foreground and address the needs of disadvantaged populations. [5]

8.3 The Joint Commission National Patient Safety Goal on Health Equity

In 2022, The Joint Commission established a **National Patient Safety Goal to Improve Health Care Equity**, recognizing that health care disparities are primarily a quality-of-care problem. [6]

Key requirements:

1. **Identify a leader** responsible for health equity efforts.
2. **Assess health-related social needs (HRSN)** for a representative sample of patients.
3. **Stratify key quality and safety measures** by patient characteristics (race, ethnicity, language, socioeconomic status)
4. **Develop a plan** to address at least one identified disparity.

Why this matters for residents:

- Your hospital is now required to measure and address disparities.
- You will see quality dashboards stratified by race, ethnicity, and language.
- You may be asked to participate in equity-focused QI projects.
- Understanding these requirements will help you lead change.

The Joint Commission's rationale:
"Although health care disparities are often viewed through the lens of social injustice, they are first and foremost a quality-of-care problem. Like medication errors, health care-acquired infections, and falls, health care disparities must be examined, the root causes understood, and the causes addressed with targeted interventions in order to improve health outcomes for all." [6]

8.4 The Health Equity Implementation Framework (HEIF)

The **Health Equity Implementation Framework (HEIF)** integrates implementation science with healthcare disparities research to provide a comprehensive approach to understanding and addressing equity in implementation. [7]

The HEIF adds three equity-focused domains to traditional implementation frameworks: [7-8]

1. The Clinical Encounter

- Patient-provided communication
- Shared decision-making
- Trust and rapport
- Implicit bias
- Cultural humility

2. Societal Context

- Structural racism
- Socioeconomic factors
- Historical trauma
- Discrimination
- Power dynamics

3. Culturally Relevant Factors

- Healthy beliefs and practices
- Language and communication preferences
- Family and community structures
- Religious and spiritual considerations
- Immigration status and acculturation

How to apply for the HEIF in your QI project: [8-9]

Step 1: Assess the clinical encounter.

- How do patients from divergent backgrounds experience care in your setting?
- Are there communication barriers (language, health literacy, cultural differences)?
- Is there evidence of implicit bias in how care is delivered?

Step 2: Assess societal context.

- What structural factors affect your patient population (housing, food security, transportation, employment)?
- How does historical discrimination affect trust in the healthcare system?

- What policies or systems create barriers to care?

Step 3: Assess culturally relevant factors.

- What are the health beliefs and practices of your patient population?
- How do family and community structures affect health decisions?
- What cultural adaptations are needed for your intervention?

Example application:
A resident is implementing a heart failure discharge bundle at a safety-net hospital serving a Black and Hispanic population.

Clinical encounter assessment:

- Many patients report feeling rushed during discharge education.
- Spanish interpreter services are not consistently used as needed.
- Some patients express distrust of the healthcare system.

Societal context assessment:

- Many patients lack transportation for follow-up appointments.
- Food insecurity makes low-sodium diet recommendations impractical.
- Historical experiences of discrimination affect willingness to engage with care.

Culturally relevant factors assessment:

- Extended family members are often involved in care decisions.
- Some patients prefer to discuss health with community health workers rather than physicians.
- Religious beliefs influence end-of-life care preferences.

Adaptations based on assessment:

- Extend discharge education time and use teach-back consistently.
- Mandate interpreter use for all non-English-speaking patients.
- Partner with health workers for post-discharge follow-up
- Provide transportation vouchers for follow-up appointments.
- Adapt dietary recommendations to be culturally appropriate and affordable.
- Include family members in discharge education.

8.5 Measuring Implementation Outcomes with an Equity Lens

Every implementation science study designed to advance health equity must define a health equity measure to evaluate the success of implementation strategies. [3]

Applying RE-AIM with an equity lens: [3] [10-12]
The RE-AIM framework (Reach, Effectiveness, Adoption, Implementation, Maintenance) can be extended to incorporate equity considerations at each dimension:

The following figure illustrates how equity considerations intersect with the RE-AIM framework at both individual and setting levels. [12]

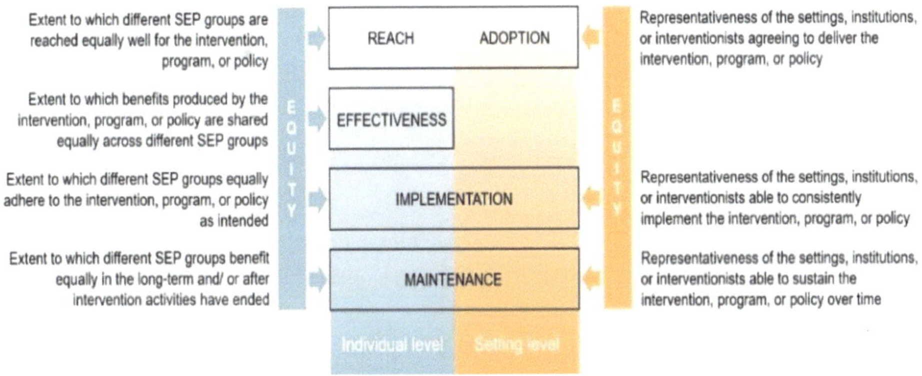

Individual- and setting-level indicators of socio-economic equity.
Copyright © 2025 the authors.
Socio-economic equity in the impact of population-based interventions to reduce alcohol consumption. Cochrane Database Syst Rev. May 6, 2025.

Reach with an equity lens:

- **Standard measure:** What percentage of eligible patients received the intervention?
- **Equity measure:** What percentage of patients from underrepresented racial and ethnic groups received the intervention? Is the reach equitable across groups? [3]
- **Equity question:** Are we reaching the patients who need this intervention most, or are we preferentially reaching those who are already advantaged?

Effectiveness with an equity lens:

- **Standard measure:** Did the intervention improve outcomes?
- **Equity measure:** Did the intervention improve outcomes equally across groups? Did it reduce, maintain, or widen disparities?
- **Equity question:** Is the intervention equally effective for all patients, or does it work better for some groups than others?

Adoption with an equity lens:

- **Standard measure:** What percentage of eligible providers/sites adopted the intervention?
- **Equity measure:** Did providers/sites serving underrepresented populations adopt the intervention at equal rates?
- **Equity question:** Are safety-net hospitals, community health centers, and providers serving marginalized populations adopting this intervention?

Implementation with an equity lens:

- **Standard measure:** Was the intervention delivered with fidelity?
- **Equity measure:** Was fidelity equal across settings serving different populations? Were adaptations made to improve equity?
- **Equity question:** Are we implementing this intervention with the same quality in under-resourced settings as in well-resourced settings?

Maintenance with an equity lens:

- **Standard measure:** Was the intervention sustained over time?

- **Equity measure:** Was sustainability equal across settings? Do under-resourced settings have the capacity to maintain the intervention?
- **Equity question:** Will this intervention be sustained in the settings that need it most, or will it fade when external support ends?

Types of health equity measures: [3]

1. **Data infrastructure measures:** Consistency in how data are captured and defined (e.g., race and ethnicity)
2. **Process and outcome measures stratified by subpopulation:** (e.g., receipt of cardiac rehabilitation stratified by racial and ethnic group)
3. **Process and outcome measures targeted at specific subpopulations:** (e.g., receipt of cardiac rehabilitation among Black patients with heart failure)
4. **Process and outcome measures targeted at strategies intended to reduce inequities:** (e.g., effectiveness of community health worker intervention in reducing readmissions among Hispanic patients)

8.6 Designing Equity-Focused QI Projects: A Practical Approach

Step 1: Stratify your baseline data.

Before embarking on QI work, examine your metric of interest by patient characteristics, starting with race and ethnicity, language, and markers of access to care and socioeconomic status. [13]

Questions to ask:

- Is there a disparity in this outcome by race, ethnicity, language, insurance status, or neighborhood?
- Which population has the worst outcomes?
- What is the magnitude of the disparity?

Example: You want to reduce the 30-day deadline for heart failure. Before designing your intervention, you stratify baseline data:

- Overall readmission rate: 25%
- White patients: 22%
- Black patients: 31%
- Hispanic patients: 28%
- Medicaid patients: 32%
- Commercially insured patients: 18%

You identify that Black patients and Medicaid patients have the highest readmission rates. Your intervention should be designed to be most effective for these populations.

Step 2: Engage stakeholders from affected communities.
Developing an understanding of existing disparities relevant to the QI project will ensure that the QI interventions can be designed to be most effective in the disadvantaged populations. [13]

Who to engage:

- Patients from the affected population
- Community health workers
- Social workers
- Community organizations
- Frontline staff who serve the affected population

What to ask:

- What barriers do patients face in accessing care?
- What would make this intervention work for your community?
- What adaptations are needed?
- What resources exist in the community that we can leverage?

Step 3: Design your intervention to address root causes.
Use the HEIF or similar framework to identify barriers at the clinical encounter, societal context, and culturally relevant factors levels. Design your intervention to address these barriers.

Step 4: Build equity into your measurement plan.

- Stratify all outcome measures by race, ethnicity, language, and socioeconomic status.
- Set explicit equity goals (e.g., "reduce the disparity in readmission rates between Black and White patients by 50%")
- Monitor for intervention-generated inequalities.

Step 5: Use Equity and Performance Improvement Toolkit

The Montefiore Center for Performance Improvement developed a novel QI toolkit that ingrains issues of diversity, equity, inclusion (DEI) and social determinants of health (SDOH) into the Institute for Healthcare Improvement's tools. [14]

Key additions to standard QI tools:

- **Updated charter:** Includes equity goals and stakeholder engagement from affected communities.
- **Stratified baseline tool:** Requires stratification of baseline data by race, ethnicity, and socioeconomic status.
- **New fishbone diagram:** Includes a "tail" for DEI and SDOH factors.
- **Updated PDSA worksheet:** Includes prompts to consider equity in Study and Act phases.

Results: After implementing this toolkit, the percentage of QI projects incorporating DEI/SDOH increased from 22.9% to 88.9%. [14]

8.7 Participatory Implementation Science

Participatory approaches to implementation science offer an inclusive, collaborative, and iterative perspective on implementing and sustaining evidence-based interventions to advance health equity. [15]

Core principles: [15]

1. **Co-production of knowledge:** Academic researchers, community members, implementers, and other actors collaboratively integrate practice-, community-, and research-based evidence.

2. **Power sharing:** Community partners are not just consulted but are true partners in decision-making.
3. **Transformational change:** The goal is not just to make interventions work within harmful systems, but to reshape systems to center equity.
4. **Bidirectional learning:** Researchers learn from communities, and communities learn from researchers.

How to apply participatory approaches in your QI project:

Engage early: Involve community partners from the beginning, not just at the end for feedback.

Share power: Give community partners real decision-making authority, not just advisory roles.

Value community expertise: Recognize that community members have knowledge that researchers lack.

Build capacity: Invest in training and resources for community partners.

Sustain relationships: Maintain partnerships beyond the project period.

Example: A residency program wants to improve diabetes control in a Hispanic community.

Traditional approach:

- Researchers design intervention based on literature.
- Implement in community health center.
- Evaluating outcomes
- Publish results.

Participatory approach:

- Researchers meet with community advisory board to understand priorities.
- Community members identify barriers (transportation, food insecurity, language, distrust)

- Community health workers are hired and trained as co-investigators.
- Intervention is co-designed with community input (Promotora model, culturally adapted education, community cooking classes)
- Community members participate in data collection and interpretation.
- Results are shared with community before publication.
- Community partners co-author publications
- Partnership continues beyond the project.

8.8 Four Principles for Equity-Focused Implementation Science

A recent narrative review identified four principles that should guide implementation science to improve equity: [3]

Principle 1: Racism must be recognized as a fundamental driver of inequities.

- Structural racism creates and maintains health disparities.
- Implementation strategies must address racism, not just its downstream effects.
- Antiracism interventions should be part of the implementation toolkit.

Principal 2: Improved equity requires engagement of community members and other relevant partners.

- Community partners should be involved from study inception to evaluation.
- Multilevel stakeholders should participate in design, execution, and policy development.
- Community expertise is essential for understanding context and designing adaptations.

Principle 3: Equitable healthcare requires multi-sector partnerships.

- Health outcomes are shaped by factors outside the healthcare system.
- Implementation strategies should connect to housing, education, employment, and other sectors.
- Cross-sector collaboration is essential for addressing social determinants.

Principle 4: Context is central to healthcare equity.

- Implementation strategies must be adapted to the local context.
- What works in one setting may not work in another?
- Understanding context requires qualitative methods and community engagement.

8.9 Data Parity in Public Health

Achieving health equity requires attention to **data equity**—ensuring that data collection, analysis, interpretation, and translation are conducted in ways that promote fairness and do not perpetuate bias. [16]

The following figure from Wang et al. illustrates a framework for promoting data equity in public health research and practice, integrating principles from both computer science (fairness, accountability, transparency, ethics, privacy) and public health (selection bias, representativeness, generalizability, causality, information bias). [16]

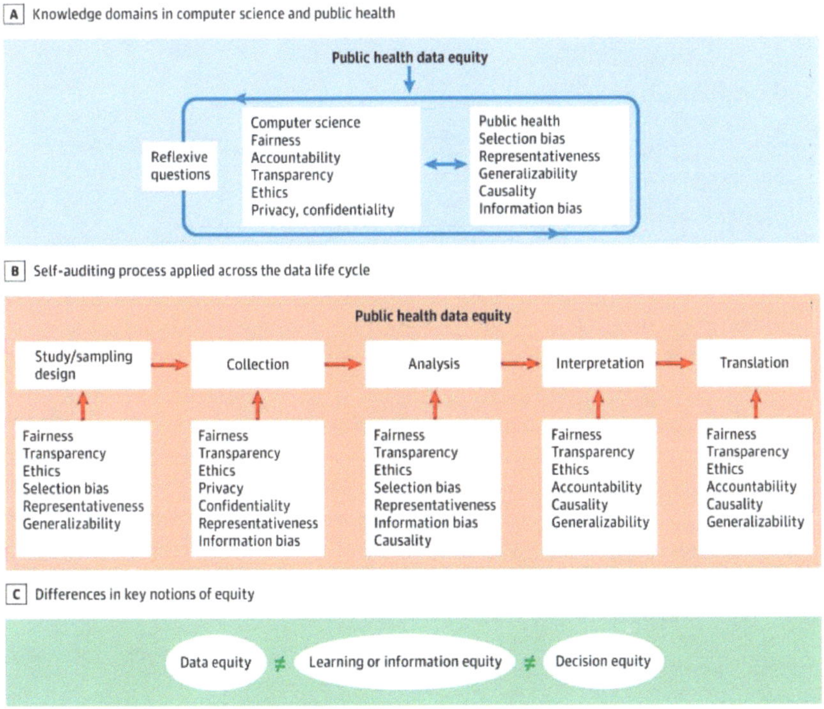

Framework for Promoting Data Equity in Public Health Research and Practice
Ten Core Concepts for Ensuring Data Equity in Public Health.
JAMA Health Forum. January 1, 2026.

Key concepts: [16]

Data equity ≠ Information equity ≠ Decision equity

- **Data equity:** Fair and unbiased data collection and analysis
- **Information equity:** Equitable dissemination of findings to all communities
- **Decision equity:** Empowering communities with decision-making agency about their health

Even when data equity is achieved, this does not automatically translate into equitable information dissemination or equitable health decision-making. Data equity is necessary but not sufficient for health equity.

Practical implications for your QI project:

- Ensure your data collection captures race, ethnicity, language, and socioeconomic status accurately and consistently.
- Stratify your analyses by these variables.
- Consider who is missing from your data (selection bias)
- Share your findings with the communities you serve, not just academic audiences.
- Involve community members in interpreting and acting on data.

8.10 Integrating Parity into Your Residency QI Project: A Checklist

Use this checklist to ensure your QI project incorporates equity:

Planning Phase:

☐ Stratified baseline data by race, ethnicity, language, insurance status, and socioeconomic indicators
☐ Identified which population has the worst outcomes
☐ Engaged stakeholders from the affected population in project design
☐ Used an equity-focused framework (HEIF, IM4Equity or similar) to assess barriers
☐ Set explicit equity goals (not just overall improvement goals)

Design Phase:

☐ Designed an intervention to address barriers faced by the most disadvantaged population
☐ Made cultural adaptations based on community input
☐ Addressed social determinants of health (transportation, food, housing, etc.)
☐ Ensured intervention is accessible to patients with limited English proficiency, low health literacy, and limited digital access
☐ Included community health workers, patient navigators, or other trusted messengers

Implementation Phase:

☐ Monitored reach by race, ethnicity, and socioeconomic status
☐ Tracked fidelity across different settings and populations
☐ Made adaptations based on feedback from affected communities
☐ Addressed barriers as they emerged

Evaluation Phase:

☐ Stratified all outcome measures by race, ethnicity, language, and socioeconomic status
☐ Assessed whether disparities were reduced, maintained, or widened
☐ Evaluated sustainability in under-resourced settings
☐ Shared results with community partners
☐ Identified lessons learned for future equity-focused work

Dissemination Phase:

☐ Shared findings with the communities served, not just academic audiences
☐ Included community partners as co-authors on publications
☐ Advocated for policy changes based on findings
☐ Sustained partnerships beyond the project period

Key Takeaways for Section 8:

✓ **Health equity should be central to every implementation project.** As a minimum, ensure that existing disparities are not widened and that no population is left behind. [1]

✓ **QI projects can worsen disparities** if not designed with equity in mind. Intervention-generated inequalities occur when improvements benefit advantaged populations more than disadvantaged populations. [4-5]

✓ **The Joint Commission now requires** hospitals to identify a health equity leader, assess health-related social needs, stratify quality measures, and develop plans to address disparities. [6]

✓ **The Health Equity Implementation Framework (HEIF)** adds three equity-focused domains to traditional implementation frameworks: the clinical encounter, societal context, and culturally relevant factors. [7-8]

✓ **Apply RE-AIM with an equity lens** by asking whether reach, effectiveness, adoption, implementation, and maintenance are equitable across populations. [3][10][12]

✓ **Stratify your baseline data** before designing your intervention to understand existing disparities and design interventions that will be most effective for disadvantaged populations. [13]

✓ **Engage community partners** as true partners in design, implementation, and evaluation—not just as advisory voices. [15]

✓ **Four principles guide equity-focused implementation:** recognize racism as a driver of inequities, engage community partners, build multisector partnerships, and address context. [3]

✓ **Data equity is necessary but not sufficient** for health equity. Equitable data practices must be accompanied by equitable information dissemination and community decision-making power. [16]

CHAPTER 9

Sustainability and Scaling

One of the most frustrating experiences in quality improvement is watching a successful intervention fade away after the initial project ends. **Like many organizational changes, quality improvement projects often experience a decline after implementation.** This phenomenon, sometimes called "improvement evaporation," occurs when the energy, attention, and resources that drove initial success are redirected elsewhere, and the intervention gradually returns to baseline. [1]

As a senior medical student or resident, understanding how to design for sustainability from the beginning—and how to scale successful interventions beyond your initial pilot—will distinguish your QI work from the many well-intentioned projects that fail to create lasting change.

9.1 Understanding Sustainability: Why Improvements Fade

Sustainability refers to the degree to which an intervention is maintained over time after external support ends. In the RE-AIM framework, this is captured in the "Maintenance" dimension, which measures how strategies were implemented beyond the predefined study period. [2]

Why have improvements faded?
A systematic integrative review of 124 studies on healthcare program sustainability identified the most common barriers and facilitators: [3]

Most common barriers to sustainability:

- **Staffing and turnover** (40.3% of studies): When champions leave, institutional memory is lost.

- **Lack of training/support/supervision** (43.5%): Skills decay without ongoing reinforcement
- **Insufficient leadership support** (49.2%): Competing priorities divert attention.
- **Funding constraints** (56.5% of studies reporting outer setting factors): Grant funding ends, and no sustainable funding source is identified.
- **Poor fit with existing systems** (reported in discontinued programs): The intervention never became integrated into routine workflow.

Most common facilitators of sustainability:

- **Strong leadership and champions** (49.2%): Visible, ongoing commitment from leaders
- **Adequate training and support** (43.5%): Continuous skill development and reinforcement
- **Integration into existing systems** (institutionalization): The intervention becomes "the way we do things."
- **Ongoing monitoring and feedback** (process factors): Data continues to drive improvement.
- **External stakeholder support** (34.8%): Alignment with external policies and guidelines

Key insight: Factors related to the inner setting (organizational context), process (how implementation is conducted), and intervention characteristics were most frequently reported as influencing sustainability. [3] This means that sustainability is not just about the intervention itself, it is about how well the intervention fits into the organizational context and how the implementation process is designed.

9.2 The QUERI Implementation Roadmap: A Framework for Sustainability

The **Quality Enhancement Research Initiative (QUERI) Implementation Roadmap**, developed by the VA health system, provides a systematic approach to planning for sustainability from the beginning of an implementation effort. [4]

The three phases of the QUERI Roadmap: [4]

Phase 1: Pre-implementation

- Identify a high-priority need.
- Select evidence-based practices (EBPs) to address the need.
- Engage stakeholders to build implementation capacity.
- Specify needed adaptations and evaluation goals.
- Activate leadership support.

Phase 2: Implementation

- Use implementation strategies to promote technical competency and adaptive skills.
- Motivate providers to own and sustain EBPs.
- Monitor fidelity and adaptation!
- Build local capacity for ongoing improvement.

Phase 3: Sustainment

- Conduct evaluation analyses that establish the business case.
- Hand off to system leadership to own implementation maintenance over time.
- Integrate the intervention into routine operations.
- Continuing monitoring and adaptation

Key insight: The Roadmap emphasizes that **sustainment is not a separate phase that happens after implementation must be planned for from the beginning.** The pre-implementation phase should include explicit planning for how the intervention will be sustained, and the implementation phase should build the capacity and ownership needed for long-term maintenance.

9.3 Building the Business Case for Sustainability

One of the most critical elements of sustainability is establishing the business case—demonstrating that the intervention provides sufficient value to justify ongoing investment of resources. [4]

Components of a business case:

1. Clinical outcomes:

- Improved patient outcomes (mortality, morbidity, quality of life)
- Reduced complications or adverse events
- Improved patient satisfaction

2. Operational outcomes:

- Improved efficiency (reduced length of stay, faster throughput)
- Reduced waste (unnecessary tests, procedures, medications)
- Improved staff satisfaction and reduced burnout

3. Financial outcomes:

- Cost savings (reduced readmissions, complications, resource use)
- Revenue enhancement (improved quality metrics, value-based payments)
- Avoided costs (prevented adverse events, litigation)

4. Strategic outcomes:

- Alignment with organizational priorities
- Competitive advantage
- Regulatory compliance
- Reputation and accreditation

The following figure illustrates the multiple domains of value that institutional leaders consider when evaluating investments in improvement programs, extending beyond simple financial return on investment. [5]

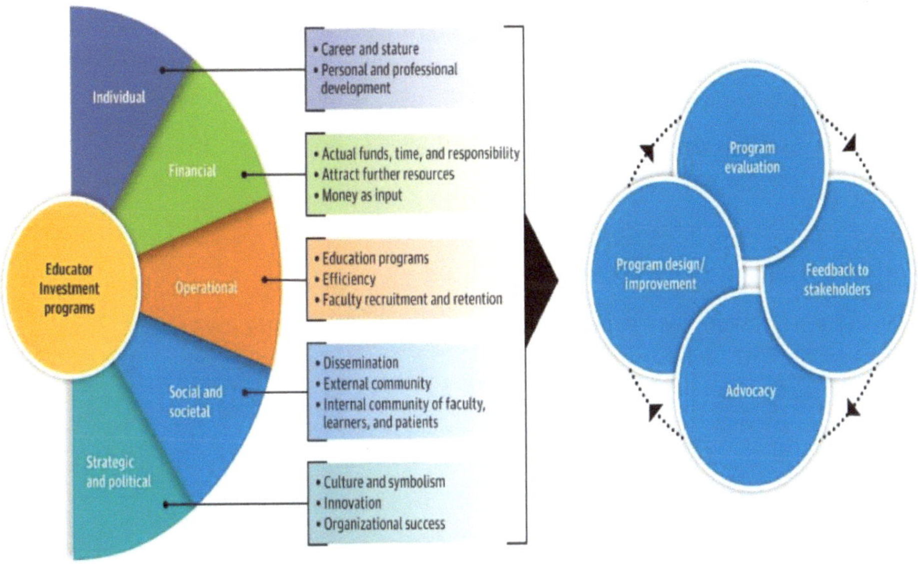

Fig. 9.3 Value domains and identified value factors

Source: Identifying Value Factors in Institutional Leaders' Perspectives on Investing in Health Professions Educators. JAMA New Open. January 31, 2023.

How to build your business case:

Step 1: Quantify the problem.

- How many patients are affected?
- What are the current outcomes?
- What are the costs of the current state (direct costs, indirect costs, opportunity costs)?

Step 2: Quantify the improvement.

- What outcomes improved?
- By how much?
- How many patients benefited?

Step 3: Calculate the value.

- What are the cost savings?
- What are the revenue implications?
- What are the intangible benefits (patient satisfaction, staff morale, reputation)?

Step 4: Compare costs.

- What does it cost to sustain the intervention (staff time, materials, technology)?
- What is the return on investment?

Step 5: Present to leadership

- Frame the business case in terms that resonate with leadership priorities.
- Use data and stories to make the case compelling.
- Propose a sustainable funding model.

9.4 Strategies for Sustaining Improvement

A scoping review of knowledge translation strategies for sustainability identified the most commonly used approaches: [6]

Most common strategies for sustainability:

1. Train and educate stakeholders

- Ongoing education for unfamiliar staff
- Refresher training for existing staff
- Integration into orientation and onboarding
- Competency assessment and feedback

2. Develop stakeholder interrelationships

- Build networks of champions across units.
- Create communities of practice.
- Foster peer-to-peer learning
- Engage patients and families as partners.

3. Audit and feedback

- Continue monitoring key metrics.
- Provide regular feedback to frontline staff.
- Celebrating successes and address gaps
- Use data to drive ongoing improvement.

4. Integrate into systems and workflows

- Embed the intervention into EHR workflows.
- Create standing orders and order sets.
- Modify policies and procedures.
- Make the desired behavior the default.

5. Engage leadership

- Maintain visible leadership support.
- Include metrics in leadership dashboards.
- Aligning with organizational strategic priorities
- Secure ongoing resource commitment

Key insight: Many studies did not clearly report whether they used different or the same strategies between implementation and sustainability phases. Only two studies reported using a new strategy specifically for sustainability, and seven studies adapted strategies from implementation to sustainability. [6] This suggests that **sustainability requires intentional, ongoing effort—not just a continuation of initial implementation activities.**

9.5 The Four Steps of Scaling Up

Scaling up refers to the process of expanding a successful intervention from a pilot site to broader implementation across multiple sites, populations, or systems. The Institute for Healthcare Improvement (IHI) framework describes four sequential steps: [7]

Step 1: Set-Up

- Prepare the ground for introduction and testing.
- Identify the problem and the evidence-based intervention.

- Engage leadership and secure commitment.
- Establish the infrastructure for scale-up.
- Define the scalable unit (the smallest unit of organization where the intervention can be successfully implemented)

Step 2: Develop the Scalable Unit

- Evaluate the intervention in a single unit or site.
- Refine the intervention based on learning.
- Develop implementation tools (protocols, training materials, data collection systems)
- Demonstrate success in the scalable unit.
- Document what works and what does not.

Step 3: Test of Scale-Up

- Evaluate the intervention in a variety of settings.
- Include settings that represent different contexts (urban/rural, large/small, high-resource/low-resource)
- Identify adaptations needed for different contexts.
- Develop strategies for addressing common barriers.
- Build capacity for broader implementation.

Step 4: Go to Full Scale

- Rapidly expand to a larger number of sites
- Use adoption mechanisms (training, technical assistance, learning collaboratives)
- Monitor implementation and outcomes across sites.
- Continue to adapt and improve.
- Institutionalize the intervention.

Key insight: The framework emphasizes the crucial importance of **defining a scalable unit of organization.** If a scalable unit can be defined, and successful results achieved by implementing an intervention in this unit without major addition of resources, it is more likely that the intervention can be fully and rapidly scaled. [7]

9.6 Factors That Facilitate and Hinder Scale-Up

A scoping review of factors affecting scale-up identified the most common facilitators and barriers: [8]

Facilitators of scale-up:

- **Strong leadership:** Committed leaders who champion the intervention.
- **Well-defined roles:** Clear responsibilities for implementation
- **Good coordination:** Effective communication and collaboration across sites
- **Positive political environment:** Alignment with policy priorities
- **Community support and engagement:** Buy-in from patients and communities.
- **Adequate resources:** Sufficient funding, staffing, and infrastructure
- **Evidence of effectiveness:** Demonstrated impact on pilot sites.

Barriers to scale-up:

- **Poor user organization:** Lack of capacity at implementing sites.
- **Unfavorable institutional environment:** Organizational culture resistance to change.
- **Inadequate resource mobilization:** Insufficient funding or staffing
- **Complexity of the intervention:** Interventions that are difficult to implement.
- **Lack of adaptation:** Failure to tailor the intervention to local context
- **Insufficient monitoring:** Lack of data to guide scale-up decisions.

Key insight: Hindering and favoring factors do not exist in isolation, but are correlated, interact, and enhance or hinder one another. [8] Successful scale-up requires attention to multiple factors simultaneously.

9.7 Evaluating Scale-Up Success

A methodological review proposed four main dimensions of scale-up success: [9]

1. Coverage: The proportion of organizations implementing the intervention

- How many sites have adopted the intervention?
- What percentage of eligible sites are implemented?

2. Reach: The proportion of the target population reached

- How many patients are receiving the intervention?
- What percentage of eligible patients are reached?

3. Effectiveness: The impact of the intervention on scale

- Are outcomes improving across sites?
- Is effectiveness maintained as the intervention scales?
- Is there variation across subgroups, providers, or regions?

4. Institutionalization: The integration of intervention into existing systems

- Is the intervention embedded in policies and procedures?
- Is it part of routine workflow?
- Will it continue without external support?

Additional considerations:

- **Cost of scale-up:** Resources required for expansion.
- **Adoption:** Decisions and actions to implement
- **Fidelity:** Adherence to the intervention as designed
- **Adaptations:** Modifications made for local context

Key insight: Longitudinal, adaptive, and mixed-methods designs are needed to capture real-world implementation dynamics during scale-up. [9] Scale-up is an iterative and adaptive process, not a linear progression.

9.8 Designing for Sustainability and Scale from the Start

The following figure from Van Spall et al. illustrates the multilevel considerations needed when designing interventions with end-of-trial implementation in mind, showing how sustainability and scalability should be considered from the earliest stages of intervention development. [10]

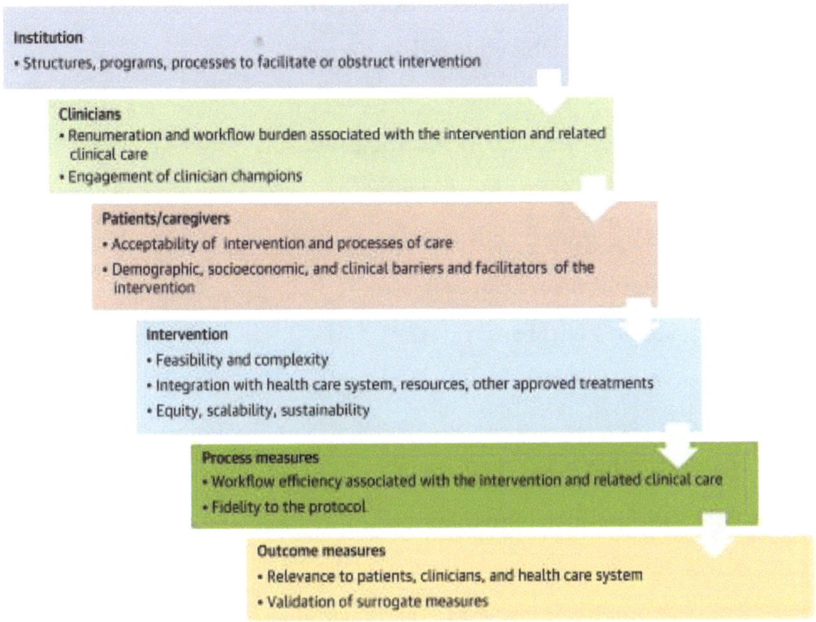

Fig. 9.2 Considerations in designing a phase 3 trial to foster end-of-trial implementation

Source: A Guide to Implementation Science for Phase 3 Clinical Trialists: Designing Trials for Evidence Uptake. J Am Coll Cardiol. November 11, 2024.

Key design considerations for sustainability and scale: [10-11]

At the institutional level:

- What structures, programs, and processes may facilitate or obstruct intervention delivery?
- How does the intervention fit with existing systems?
- What infrastructure is needed for long-term maintenance?

At the clinician level:

- What are the workflow burdens associated with the intervention?
- How will clinicians be trained and supported?
- Who will champion the intervention?

At the patient/caregiver level:

- Is the intervention acceptable to patients?
- What demographic, socioeconomic, and clinical barriers exist?
- How will patients be engaged as partners?

At the intervention level:

- Is intervention feasible in routine practice?
- How complex is it to implement?
- Can it be integrated with existing resources?
- Is it equitable across populations?
- Is it scalable to other settings?
- Is it sustainable without external support?

Process measures:

- How will workflow efficiency be monitored?
- How will fidelity to the intervention be assessed?

Outcome measures:

- Are outcomes relevant to patients, clinicians, and health systems?
- How will effectiveness be measured on a scale?

9.9 The Implementability Framework: Acceptability, Fidelity, Feasibility, Scalability, Sustainability

An overview of reviews proposed a conceptual framework of **implementability** that links five key concepts: [11]

Acceptability: The perception among stakeholders that the intervention is agreeable or satisfactory.

- Do patients, clinicians, and leaders support the intervention?
- Is it consistent with values and preferences?

Fidelity: The degree to which the intervention is delivered as intended.

- Are core components being implemented correctly?
- What adaptations are being made?

Feasibility: The extent to which the intervention can be successfully conducted

- Can it be delivered with available resources?
- Does it fit into existing workflows?

Scalability: The ability to expand the intervention to reach more people or settings

- Can it be replicated in other contexts?
- What adaptations are needed for different settings?

Sustainability: The extent to which the intervention is maintained over time

- Will it continue after external support ends?
- Is it integrated into routine practice?

Key insight: The expert panel proposed that **scalability and sustainability are dependent on acceptability, fidelity, and feasibility.** Furthermore, these factors require re-evaluation over time and as the intervention is implemented in different settings or with different populations. [11]

Practical implication: Before attempting to scale or sustain an intervention, assess whether it is acceptable, feasible, and being implemented with fidelity. If these foundational elements are not in place, scale-up and sustainability efforts are likely to fail.

9.10 Practical Strategies for Your Residency QI Project

Planning for sustainability from the start:

☐ **Engage leadership early:** Secure visible commitment from department and hospital leadership

☐ **Build a coalition of champions:** Identify and engage frontline staff who will own the intervention

☐ **Integrate into existing systems:** Design the intervention to fit into current workflows, EHR systems, and policies

☐ **Plan for staff turnover:** Develop training materials and onboarding processes for unfamiliar staff

☐ **Establish ongoing monitoring:** Create dashboards and feedback mechanisms that will continue after the project ends

☐ **Build the business case:** Document outcomes and costs to justify ongoing investment

☐ **Plan the handoff:** Identify who will own the intervention after you leave

Designing for scale:

☐ **Define the scalable unit:** What is the smallest unit where the intervention can succeed?

☐ **Document what works:** Create implementation guides, protocols, and training materials

☐ **Test in diverse settings:** If possible, pilot in settings that represent different contexts

☐ **Identify adaptations:** Document what modifications are needed for different settings

☐ **Build capacity:** Train others to implement and spread the intervention

☐ **Engage stakeholders:** Build relationships with leaders and champions at potential scale-up sites

Common pitfalls to avoid:

✗ **Treating sustainability as an afterthought:** Plan for sustainability from day one

✗ **Relying on a single champion:** Build a coalition so the intervention survives turnover

✗ **Failing to integrate into systems:** Interventions that require extra work will fade

✗ **Not building the business case:** Without demonstrated value, resources will be redirected

✗ **Assuming one size fits all:** Adaptations are needed for different contexts

✗ **Stopping monitoring too soon:** Ongoing data is needed to maintain gains

9.11 Case Example: Sustaining a Heart Failure Discharge Bundle

The intervention: A resident-led QI project implemented a heart failure discharge bundle including medication reconciliation, patient education, follow-up appointment scheduling, and post-discharge phone calls. **Initial results:** 30-day readmission rate decreased from 28% to 19%.

Sustainability challenges:

- The resident who led the project graduated
- The nurse who made post-discharge calls was reassigned.
- Competing priorities diverted attention.
- Readmission rates began to creep back up.

Sustainability strategies implemented:

1. **Integrated into EHR:** Created a heart failure discharge order set that automatically triggered the bundle components.
2. **Built into workflow:** Made the discharge checklist part of the standard discharge process for all heart failure patients.
3. **Trained multiple staff:** Cross-trained several nurses to make post-discharge calls.
4. **Established ongoing monitoring:** Created a monthly dashboard reviewed at department meetings.
5. **Built the business case:** Documented cost savings from reduced readmissions ($15,000 per avoided readmission × 20 avoided readmissions = $300,000 annual savings)
6. **Secured leadership commitment:** Presented results to hospital leadership, who committed ongoing resources.
7. **Handed off to a permanent champion:** Identified a hospitalist faculty member to own the program long-term.

Outcome: Readmission rates remained at 20% two years after the initial project, with the intervention fully integrated into routine care.

Key Takeaways for Section 9:

✓ **QI projects frequently decline after implementation.** Sustainability must be planned from the beginning, not treated as an afterthought. [1][3]

✓ **The QUERI Implementation Roadmap** provides a systematic approach with three phases: pre-implementation, implementation, and sustainment. The sustainment phase includes establishing the business case and handing off to system leadership. [4]

✓ **Building the business case** is critical for sustainability. Demonstrate value across clinical, operational, financial, and strategic domains to justify ongoing investment. [5]

✓ **Key strategies for sustainability** include ongoing training, stakeholder engagement, audit and feedback, integration into systems, and continued leadership support. [3][6]

✓ **Scaling up follows four steps:** Set-up, develop the scalable unit, test of scale-up, and go to full scale. Defining a scalable unit is crucial. [7]

✓ **Scale-up success** is measured by coverage, reach, effectiveness, and institutionalization, contingent on cost, adoption, fidelity, and adaptations. [9]

✓ **Scalability and sustainability depend on acceptability, fidelity, and feasibility.** Assess these foundational elements before attempting to scale or sustain. [11]

✓ **Design for sustainability and scale from the start** by engaging leadership, building coalitions, integrating into systems, planning for turnover, establishing monitoring, and building the business case. [10]

One of the most frustrating experiences in quality improvement is watching a successful intervention fade away after the initial project ends. **Like many organizational changes, quality improvement projects often experience a decline after implementation.** This phenomenon, sometimes called "improvement evaporation," occurs when the energy, attention, and resources that drove initial success are redirected elsewhere, and the intervention gradually returns to baseline. [1]

As a senior medical student or resident, understanding how to design for sustainability from the beginning—and how to scale successful interventions beyond your initial pilot—will distinguish your QI work from the many well-intentioned projects that fail to create lasting change.

References

1. The Academic Learning Health System: A Framework for Integrating the Multiple Missions of Academic Medical Centers. Academic Medicine: Journal of the Association of American Medical Colleges. 2023. Rosenthal GE, McClain DA, High KP, et al.
2. Bridging Treatment Implementation Gaps in Patients with Heart Failure: JACC Focus Seminar 2/3. Journal of the American College of Cardiology. 2023. Jalloh MB, Averbuch T, Kulkarni P, et al.
3. Implementation Science to Achieve Equity in Heart Failure Care: A Scientific Statement from the American Heart Association. Circulation. 2024. Breathett K, Lewsey S, Brownell NK, et al.
4. Competences for Implementation Science: What Trainees Need to Learn and Where They Learn It. Advances in Health Sciences Education: Theory and Practice. 2021. Schultes MT, Aijaz M, Klug J, Fixsen DL.
5. A Framework for Training Health Professionals in Implementation and Dissemination Science. Academic Medicine: Journal of the Association of American Medical Colleges. 2012. Gonzales R, Handley MA, Ackerman S, O'sullivan PS.
6. Revolutionized Public Health Teaching to Equip Medical Students for 21st Century Practice. American Journal of Preventive Medicine. 2020. Shaw CV, D'Souza AJ, Cunningham R, Sarfati D.
7. Quality Improvement Education for Medical Students: A Near-Peer Pilot Study. BMC Medical Education. 2020. McGeorge E, Coughlan C, Fawcett M, Klaber RE.
8. How Can Medical Students Add Value? Identifying Roles, Barriers, and Strategies to Advance the Value of Undergraduate Medical Education to Patient Care and the Health System. Academic Medicine: Journal of the Association of American Medical Colleges. 2017. Gonzalo JD, Dekhtyar M, Hawkins RE, Wolpaw DR.
9. Developing a Professional Identity as a Change Agent Early in Medical School: The Students' Voice. Journal of General Internal Medicine. 2019. McDermott C, Shank K, Shervinskie C, Gonzalo JD.
10. Health Systems Science in Medical Education: Unifying the Components to Catalyze Transformation. Academic Medicine: Journal of the Association of American Medical Colleges. 2020. Gonzalo JD, Chang A, Dekhtyar M, et al.
11. Integration of Health Systems Science and Women's Healthcare. American Journal of Obstetrics and Gynecology. 2022. Morosky CM, Cox SM, Craig LB, et al.
12. Health Systems Science Curricula in Undergraduate Medical Education: Identifying and Defining a Potential Curricular Framework. Academic Medicine: Journal of the Association of American Medical Colleges. 2017. Gonzalo JD, Dekhtyar M, Starr SR, et al.

13. Socially Accountable Academic Health Centers: Pursuing a Quadripartite Mission. Academic Medicine: Journal of the Association of American Medical Colleges. 2019. Smitherman HC, Baker RS, Wilson MR.
14. Combining Patient, Clinical and System Perspectives in Assessing Performance in Healthcare: An Integrated Measurement Framework. BMC Health Services Research. 2020. Levesque JF, Sutherland K.
15. Academic Health Centers and the Quintuple Aim of Health Care. Academic Medicine: Journal of the Association of American Medical Colleges. 2023. Farrell TW, Greer AG, Bennie S, Hageman H, Pfeifle A.
16. Characteristics of Academic-Affiliated Health Systems. Academic Medicine: Journal of the Association of American Medical Colleges. 2020. Niedzwiecki MJ, Machta RM, Reschovsky JD, Furukawa MF, Rich EC.
17. Now Is Our Time to Act: Why Academic Medicine Must Embrace Community Collaboration as Its Fourth Mission. Academic Medicine: Journal of the Association of American Medical Colleges. 2021. Alberti P, Fair M, Skorton DJ.
18. Health Equity and the Tripartite Mission: Moving from Academic Health Centers to Academic-Community Health Systems. Academic Medicine: Journal of the Association of American Medical Colleges. 2019. Park B, Frank B, Likumahuwa-Ackman S, et al.
19. Creating a Quality Improvement Course for Undergraduate Medical Education: Practice What You Teach. Academic Medicine: Journal of the Association of American Medical Colleges. 2018. Bradham TS, Sponsler KC, Watkins SC, Ehrenfeld JM.
20. A Realist Synthesis of Quality Improvement Curricula in Undergraduate and Postgraduate Medical Education: What Works, for Whom, and in What Contexts? BMJ Quality & Safety. 2021. Brown A, Lafreniere K, Freedman D, et al.
21. Implementation and Evaluation of an Elective Quality Improvement Curriculum for Preclinical Students: A Prospective Controlled Study. BMC Medical Education. 2023. Aredo JV, Ding JB, Lai CH, et al.
22. Efficacy of Quality Improvement and Patient Safety Workshops for Students: A Pilot Study. BMC Medical Education. 2020. Shah KP, Goyal S, Ramachandran V, et al.
23. Evaluation of a Quality Improvement Experience for Family Medicine Clerkship Students. Family Medicine. 2021. Mills G, Kelly S, Crittendon DR, Cunningham A, Arenson C.
24. Preparing Medical Students to Incorporate Scientific Evidence into Patient Care: A Cross-Sectional Study. PloS One. 2024. Wallerstedt SM, Garwicz M, Henriksson P, et al.
25. Methods for Teaching Evidence-Based Practice: a Scoping Review. BMC Medical Education. 2019. Larsen CM, Terkelsen AS, Carlsen AF, Kristensen HK.
26. A Prospective Study Evaluating the Integration of a Multifaceted Evidence-Based Medicine Curriculum into Early Years in an Undergraduate Medical School. BMC Medical Education. 2020. Kumaravel B, Jenkins H, Chepkin S, et al.
27. Designing Evidence-Based Medicine Training to Optimize the Transfer of Skills from the Classroom to Clinical Practice: Applying the Four Component Instructional Design Model. Academic Medicine: Journal of the Association of American Medical Colleges. 2015. Maggio LA, Cate OT, Irby DM, O'Brien BC.
28. Patience, Persistence and Pragmatism: Experiences and Lessons Learnt from the Implementation of Clinically Integrated Teaching and Learning of Evidence-Based Health Care - A Qualitative Study. PloS One. 2015. Young T, Rohwer A, van Schalkwyk S, Volmink J, Clarke M.
29. Development and Evaluation of an Evidence-Based Medicine Module in the Undergraduate Medical Curriculum. BMC Medical Education. 2020. Al Shahrani AS.
30. Database Combinations to Retrieve Systematic Reviews in Overviews of Reviews: A Methodological Study. BMC Medical Research Methodology. 2020. Goossen K, Hess S, Lunny C, Pieper D.

31. The Optimal Approach for Retrieving Systematic Reviews Was Achieved When Searching for MEDLINE and Epistemonikos in Addition to Reference Checking: A Methodological Validation Study. BMC Medical Research Methodology. 2024. Heinen L, Goossen K, Lunny C, et al.
32. Sensitive Clinical Queries Retrieved Relevant Systematic Reviews as Well as Primary Studies: An Analytic Survey. Journal of Clinical Epidemiology. 2011. Wilczynski NL, McKibbon KA, Haynes RB.
33. Toolkit of Methodological Resources to Conduct Systematic Reviews. F1000Research. 2020. Roqué M, Martínez-García L, Solà I, et al.
34. Methodologies for the Development of CHEST Guidelines and Expert Panel Reports. Chest. 2014. Lewis SZ, Diekemper R, Ornelas J, Casey KR.
35. Methodological Standards for Meta-Analyses and Qualitative Systematic Reviews of Cardiac Prevention and Treatment Studies: A Scientific Statement from the American Heart Association. Circulation. 2017. Rao G, Lopez-Jimenez F, Boyd J, et al.
36. How to Interpret and Use a Clinical Practice Guideline or Recommendation: Users' Guides to Medical Literature. The Journal of the American Medical Association. 2021. Brignardello-Petersen R, Carrasco-Labra A, Guyatt GH.
37. Academic Medicine's Fourth Mission: Building Community-Oriented Primary Care to Achieve Community-Engaged Health Care. Academic Medicine: Journal of the Association of American Medical Colleges. 2023. Savage Hoggard CL, Kaufman A, Michener JL, Phillips RL.
38. Awareness, Adjustment, Assistance, Alignment, and Advocacy: Operationalizing Social Determinants of Health Topics in Undergraduate Medical Education Curricula. Academic Medicine: Journal of the Association of American Medical Colleges. 2023. Sandhu S, Solomon L, Gottlieb LM.
39. Why and How Civic Health Should Be Incorporated into Medical Education. Academic Medicine: Journal of the Association of American Medical Colleges. 2022. Barrere-Cain R, Garriga M, Kaki DA, et al.
40. Competencies for the Use of Artificial Intelligence in Primary Care. Annals of Family Medicine. 2022. Liaw W, Kueper JK, Lin S, Bazemore A, Kakadiaris I.
41. The Digital Health Competencies in Medical Education Framework: An International Consensus Statement Based on a Delphi Study. JAMA Network Open. 2025. Car J, Ong QC, Erlikh Fox T, et al.
42. Ethical Issues in Implementation Science: Perspectives from a National Heart, Lung, and Blood Institute Workshop. Implementation Science: IS. 2024. Dickert NW, Spiegelman D, Blumenthal-Barby JS, et al.
43. Making the Connection Between Health Equity and Sustainability. Frontiers in Public Health. 2023. Shelton RC, Hailemariam M, Iwelunmor J.
44. Transforming the Field: The Role of Academic Health Centers in Promoting and Sustaining Equity Based Community Engaged Research. Frontiers in Public Health. 2023. Sanchez-Youngman S, Adsul P, Gonzales A, et al.
45. Exemplary Care and Learning Sites: A Model for Achieving Continual Improvement in Care and Learning in the Clinical Setting. Academic Medicine: Journal of the Association of American Medical Colleges. 2016. Headrick LA, Ogrinc G, Hoffman KG, et al.
46. An Institutional System to Monitor and Improve the Quality of Residency Education. Academic Medicine: Journal of the Association of American Medical Colleges. 2004. Heard JK, O'Sullivan P, Smith CE, Harper RA, Schexnayder SM.
47. Using Dashboards to Support Continuous Quality Improvement in Undergraduate and Graduate Medical Education. Journal of General Internal Medicine. 2025. Dufault CL, Colson ER, Dallaghan GLB, et al.
48. Five Tactics to Quickly Build Quality Improvement and Patient Safety Capacity at Academic Health Centers. Academic Medicine: Journal of the Association of American Medical Colleges. 2017. Stevens CD.

Appendix: Quick-Reference Tools and Checklists

A Note on Visual Materials

All figures, tables, charts, and images included throughout this handbook are reproduced with appropriate academic citations indicating their original source publications. These visual materials are drawn from peer-reviewed journals including *JAMA*, *JAMA Network Open*, *New England Journal of Medicine*, *Circulation*, *Implementation Science*, *BMJ Quality & Safety*, *Cochrane Database of Systematic Reviews*, and *Journal of the American College of Cardiology*, among others. Full bibliographic information for each visual is provided in the corresponding in-text citation. Readers seeking the original context or additional details should consult the primary source publications.

A.1 Core Implementation Science Frameworks

Framework	Purpose	Key Components	When to Use	Handbook Section
RE-AIM	Planning and evaluation	Reach, Effectiveness, Adoption, Implementation, Maintenance	Planning any implementation project, evaluating outcomes	Section 4
CFIR	Assessing barriers and facilitators	Intervention, Inner Setting, Outer Setting, Individuals, Process	Diagnosing why implementation is succeeding or failing	Section 4
Model for Improve-ment	QI methodology	Three questions + PDSA cycles	Any QI project	Section 10
HEIF	Equity-focused implementation	Clinical Encounter, Societal Context, Culturally Relevant Factors	Projects serving diverse or underserved populations	Section 8

Framework	Purpose	Key Components	When to Use	Handbook Section
QUERI Roadmap	Sustainability planning	Pre-implementation, Implementation, Sustainment	Planning for long-term maintenance	Section 9
IHI Scaling Framework	Spreading interventions	Set-up, Develop Scalable Unit, Test Scale-up, Full Scale	Expanding successful pilots	Section 9

A.2 The RE-AIM Framework: Quick Reference

Dimension	Definition	Key Questions	Sample Measures
Reach	Proportion of the target population that participates	Who received the intervention? Who was missed?	% eligible patients reached; demographics of participants vs. non-participants
Effectiveness	Impact on outcomes	Did outcomes improve? For whom?	Clinical outcomes; patient-reported outcomes; adverse events
Adoption	Proportion of settings/providers that adopt	Which sites/providers implemented? Which did not?	% of eligible sites adopting; characteristics of adopters vs. non-adopters
Implementation	Fidelity and adaptations	Was it delivered as intended? What was modified?	Fidelity scores: adaptations documented; cost of delivery
Maintenance	Sustainability over time	Is it still working 6-12 months later?	Outcomes at follow-up; institutionalization; ongoing resource commitment

A.3 The CFIR Domains: Quick Reference

Domain	Definition	Example Constructs	Sample Assessment Questions
Intervention Characteristics	Features of the intervention being implemented	Evidence strength, relative advantage, complexity, adaptability	Is the intervention supported by compelling evidence? Is it better than the current practice? How complex is it?
Outer Setting	External context	Patient needs, external policies, peer pressure, incentives	What external policies support or hinder implementation? What do patients need?
Inner Setting	Organizational context	Culture, leadership, resources, readiness for change	Does leadership support this? Are resources available? Is the organization ready?
Characteristics of Individuals	People involved in implementation	Knowledge, self-efficacy, motivation	Do staff have the knowledge and skills? Are they motivated?
Process	How implementation is executed	Planning, engaging, executing, reflecting	Is there a clear plan? Are stakeholders engaged? Is progress being monitored?

A.4 The Model for Improvement: Quick Reference

Three Fundamental Questions:

1. **What are we trying to accomplish?** → Write a SMART Aim Statement
2. **How will we know that a change is an improvement?** → Define Measures (Outcome, Process, Balancing)
3. **What changes can we make that will result in improvement?** → Develop and Test Changes

The PDSA Cycle:

- **Plan:** What do you predict will happen? What data will you collect?
- **Do:** Conduct the test on a small scale. Document what happens.
- **Study:** Analyze the data. Compare results to predictions. What did you learn?
- **Act:** What will you do next? Adopt, adapt, or abandon?

PDSA Progression:
PDSA 1 → Small test (1 patient, 1 provider, 1 day)
PDSA 2 → Refine based on learning, expand slightly.
PDSA 3 → Test with more patients/providers
PDSA 4+ → Continue iterating until ready to implement broadly.

A.5 SMART Aim Statement Template

Formula:
We will [improve/increase/decrease] [specific measure] from [baseline] to [target] in [population] at [setting] by [date].

Examples:
✓ "We will increase the percentage of patients with diabetes who have HbA1c <8% from 55% to 70% in our resident continuity clinic by June 2027."

✓ "We will reduce 30-day readmission rates for heart failure patients discharged from our hospital medicine service from 25% to 18% within 12 months."

✓ "We will increase influenza vaccination rates among patients aged 65+ from 62% to 80% in our primary care practice by March 2027."

Checklist:
☐ **Specific:** What exactly will improve?
☐ **Measurable:** Can you quantify it?
☐ **Achievable:** Is the target realistic?
☐ **Relevant:** Does it matter to patients, staff, and the institution?
☐ **Time-bound:** By when?

A.6 Three Types of Measures

Measure Type	Purpose	Examples	Key Question
Outcome Measures	Did we achieve the desired result?	30-day readmission rate; HbA1c; patient satisfaction; mortality	Did the intervention work?
Process Measures	Are we implementing the intervention as intended?	% patients receiving discharge education; % orders placed correctly; % screenings completed	Are we doing what we planned?
Balancing Measures	Are there unintended consequences?	Length of stay; cost; staff workload; patient complaints; time to other care	Are we causing harm elsewhere?

A.7 Implementation Outcomes: The Proctor Taxonomy

Outcome	Definition	Sample Measures
Acceptability	Perception that the intervention is agreeable or satisfactory	Stakeholder satisfaction surveys; qualitative interviews
Adoption	Decision to employ the intervention	% of eligible providers/sites using the intervention
Appropriateness	Perceived fit for the setting and population	Stakeholder ratings of fit; alignment with needs
Feasibility	Extend to which the intervention can be conducted	Ability to deliver as intended; resource requirements
Fidelity	Degree to which the intervention is delivered as designed	Adherence to protocol; competency assessments
Implementation Cost	Resources required for implementation	Direct costs; staff time; opportunity costs

Outcome	Definition	Sample Measures
Penetration	Integration into routine practice	% of eligible patients receiving the intervention
Sustainability	Maintenance over time after external support ends	Outcomes at 6-12 months post-implementation

A.8 The Five Steps of Evidence-Based Medicine

Step	Action	Key Skills
1. ASK	Convert clinical uncertainty into an answerable question	PICO format (Patient, Intervention, Comparison, Outcome)
2. ACQUIRE	Search for the best available evidence	PubMed, Cochrane, UpToDate, clinical guidelines
3. APPRAISE	Critically evaluate the evidence	Assess validity, importance, and applicability
4. APPLY	Integrate evidence with clinical expertise and patient values	Shared decision-making; consider context
5. ASSESS	Evaluate your performance and outcomes	Reflect on the process; track outcomes

A.9 Hierarchy of Evidence

From Strongest to Weakest:

1. **Systematic reviews and meta-analyses** of randomized controlled trials
2. **Randomized controlled trials** (RCTs)
3. **Cohort studies** (prospective > retrospective)
4. **Case-control studies**
5. **Case series and case reports**
6. **Expert opinion, editorials, narrative reviews**

Remember: Higher-level evidence is not always available or applicable. Use the best available evidence for your clinical question.

A.10 Health Equity Checklist for QI Projects

Planning Phase:

☐ Stratified baseline data by race, ethnicity, language, insurance, socioeconomic status

☐ Identified which population has the worst outcomes

☐ Engaged stakeholders from the affected population

☐ Used an equity-focused framework (HEIF or similar)

☐ Set explicit equity goals

Design Phase:

☐ Designed intervention to address barriers faced by the most disadvantaged

☐ Made cultural adaptations based on community input

☐ Addressed social determinants (transportation, food, housing)

☐ Ensured accessibility for patients with limited English proficiency, low health literacy, limited digital access

☐ Included community health workers or trusted messengers

Implementation Phase:

☐ Monitored reach by race, ethnicity, socioeconomic status

☐ Tracked fidelity across different settings and populations

☐ Made adaptations based on community feedback

Evaluation Phase:

☐ Stratified all outcome measures by demographics

☐ Assessed whether disparities were reduced, maintained, or widened

☐ Shared results with community partners

A.11 Sustainability Checklist

Plan for Sustainability from Day One:

☐ Engaged leadership early and secured visible commitment
☐ Built a coalition of champions (not just one person)
☐ Integrated into existing systems (EHR, workflows, policies)
☐ Planned for staff turnover (training materials, onboarding)
☐ Established ongoing monitoring (dashboards, regular reports)
☐ Built the business case (documented outcomes and costs)
☐ Planned the handoff (identified permanent owner)

Before You Leave:

☐ Documented what works and what does not
☐ Created implementation guides and protocols
☐ Trained successors
☐ Presented results to leadership
☐ Secured ongoing resource commitment

A.12 SQUIRE 2.0 Reporting Checklist (Abbreviated)

Title: Indicate that this is a QI study

Abstract: Summarize problem, intervention, results

Introduction:

- Describe the problem and its importance.
- Summarize what is known.
- State your aim.

Methods:

- Describe the context (setting, population, culture)
- Describe the intervention(s)
- Describe measures and data collection.
- Describe analysis.

Results:

- Report outcomes with run charts/control charts.
- Describe evolution through PDSA cycles.

Discussion:

- Interpret results.
- Discuss limitations.
- Describe lessons learned.
- Discuss sustainability and spread.

A.13 Digital Health and AI: Critical Appraisal Questions

When evaluating any AI tool, ask:

1. **What problem does it solve?** Is AI the right solution?
2. **How was it developed?** What data? How validated?
3. **How does it perform?** Sensitivity, specificity, false positive rate?
4. **Is it fair?** Performance across demographic groups? Known biases?
5. **Is it explainable?** Can you understand and explain its recommendations?
6. **How does it integrate?** Fit workflow? Who acts on outputs?
7. **What's governance?** Who is accountable? How is it monitored?
8. **What are the costs?** Justified by benefits?

A.14 Telemedicine Appropriateness Quick Guide

Generally Appropriate:

- Chronic disease follow-up (stable diabetes, hypertension, heart failure)
- Mental health (therapy, medication management)
- Post-operative follow-up (wound checks, symptom assessment)
- Medication management (refills, dose adjustments)
- Patient education and counseling
- Triage (determining need for in-person evaluation)

Generally, NOT Appropriate:

- Acute emergencies (chest pain, stroke, severe dyspnea)
- Conditions requiring physical examination (new abdominal pain, new neurological symptoms)
- Procedures requiring first-hand care.
- Patients who prefer in-person care
- Situations where privacy cannot be ensured.

A.15 QI Project Timeline Template (12-18 Months)

Months 1-2: Planning

- Identify problems and team.
- Review literature and existing data.
- Map current process.
- Conduct root cause analysis.
- Write aim statement and define measures.
- Develop data collection plan.

Months 3-4: Baseline

- Collect baseline data.
- Engage stakeholders.
- Develop intervention.
- Plan first PDSA cycle.

Months 5-10: Implementation

- Conduct PDSA cycles (typically 3-5)
- Collect data continuously.
- Refine intervention based on learning.
- Address barriers as they emerge.

Months 11-12: Evaluation and Sustainability

- Analyze results.
- Document lessons learned.
- Plan for sustainability.
- Hand off to permanent owner.
- Prepare presentation/publication.

Months 13-18: Dissemination

- Present at institutional forums
- Submit to conferences.
- Write up for publication.
- Apply for MOC credit.

A.9 Hierarchy of Evidence

From Strongest to Weakest:

1. **Systematic reviews and meta-analyses** of randomized controlled trials
2. **Randomized controlled trials** (RCTs)
3. **Cohort studies** (prospective > retrospective)
4. **Case-control studies**
5. **Case series and case reports**
6. **Expert opinion, editorials, narrative reviews**

Remember: Higher-level evidence is not always available or applicable. Use the best available evidence for your clinical question.

A.10 Health Equity Checklist for QI Projects

Planning Phase:

☐ Stratified baseline data by race, ethnicity, language, insurance, socioeconomic status

☐ Identified which population has the worst outcomes

☐ Engaged stakeholders from the affected population

☐ Used an equity-focused framework (HEIF or similar)

☐ Set explicit equity goals

Design Phase:

☐ Designed intervention to address barriers faced by the most disadvantaged

☐ Made cultural adaptations based on community input

☐ Addressed social determinants (transportation, food, housing)

☐ Ensured accessibility for patients with limited English proficiency, low health literacy, limited digital access

☐ Included community health workers or trusted messengers

Implementation Phase:

☐ Monitored reach by race, ethnicity, socioeconomic status

☐ Tracked fidelity across different settings and populations

☐ Made adaptations based on community feedback

Evaluation Phase:

☐ Stratified all outcome measures by demographics

☐ Assessed whether disparities were reduced, maintained, or widened

☐ Shared results with community partners

A.11 Sustainability Checklist

Plan for Sustainability from Day One:

☐ Engaged leadership early and secured visible commitment
☐ Built a coalition of champions (not just one person)
☐ Integrated into existing systems (EHR, workflows, policies)
☐ Planned for staff turnover (training materials, onboarding)
☐ Established ongoing monitoring (dashboards, regular reports)
☐ Built the business case (documented outcomes and costs)
☐ Planned the handoff (identified permanent owner)

Before You Leave:

☐ Documented what works and what does not
☐ Created implementation guides and protocols
☐ Trained successors
☐ Presented results to leadership
☐ Secured ongoing resource commitment

A.12 SQUIRE 2.0 Reporting Checklist (Abbreviated)

Title: Indicate that this is a QI study

Abstract: Summarize problem, intervention, results

Introduction:

- Describe the problem and its importance.
- Summarize what is known.
- State your aim.

Methods:

- Describe the context (setting, population, culture)
- Describe the intervention(s)
- Describe measures and data collection.
- Describe analysis.

Results:

- Report outcomes with run charts/control charts.
- Describe evolution through PDSA cycles.

Discussion:

- Interpret results.
- Discuss limitations.
- Describe lessons learned.
- Discuss sustainability and spread.

A.13 Digital Health and AI: Critical Appraisal Questions

When evaluating any AI tool, ask:

1. **What problem does it solve?** Is AI the right solution?
2. **How was it developed?** What data? How validated?
3. **How does it perform?** Sensitivity, specificity, false positive rate?
4. **Is it fair?** Performance across demographic groups? Known biases?
5. **Is it explainable?** Can you understand and explain its recommendations?
6. **How does it integrate?** Fit workflow? Who acts on outputs?
7. **What's governance?** Who is accountable? How is it monitored?
8. **What are the costs?** Justified by benefits?

A.14 Telemedicine Appropriateness Quick Guide

Generally Appropriate:

- Chronic disease follow-up (stable diabetes, hypertension, heart failure)
- Mental health (therapy, medication management)
- Post-operative follow-up (wound checks, symptom assessment)
- Medication management (refills, dose adjustments)
- Patient education and counseling
- Triage (determining need for in-person evaluation)

Generally, NOT Appropriate:

- Acute emergencies (chest pain, stroke, severe dyspnea)
- Conditions requiring physical examination (new abdominal pain, new neurological symptoms)
- Procedures requiring first-hand care.
- Patients who prefer in-person care
- Situations where privacy cannot be ensured.

A.15 QI Project Timeline Template (12-18 Months)

Months 1-2: Planning

- Identify problems and team.
- Review literature and existing data.
- Map current process.
- Conduct root cause analysis.
- Write aim statement and define measures.
- Develop data collection plan.

Months 3-4: Baseline

- Collect baseline data.
- Engage stakeholders.
- Develop intervention.
- Plan first PDSA cycle.

Months 5-10: Implementation

- Conduct PDSA cycles (typically 3-5)
- Collect data continuously.
- Refine intervention based on learning.
- Address barriers as they emerge.

Months 11-12: Evaluation and Sustainability

- Analyze results.
- Document lessons learned
- Plan for sustainability
- Hand off to permanent owner
- Prepare presentation/publication.

Months 13-18: Dissemination

- Present at institutional forums
- Submit to conferences.
- Write up for publication.
- Apply for MOC credit.

A.16 Key Resources

Resource	What It Offers	Access
IHI Open School	Free courses on QI, patient safety, leadership	ihi.org/education
SQUIRE 2.0 Guidelines	Reporting standards for QI publications	squire-statement.org
CFIR Guide	Interactive tool for using CFIR	cfirguide.org
RE-AIM Website	Resources for applying for RE-AIM	re-aim.org
AHRQ Quality Indicators	Standardized measures for benchmarking	qualityindicators.ahrq.gov
Cochrane Library	Systematic reviews	cochranelibrary.com
UpToDate	Clinical decision support	uptodate.com
PubMed	Medical literature database	pubmed.ncbi.nlm.nih.gov
AAMC Telehealth Competencies	Framework for telehealth education	aamc.org
FDA Digital Health Center	Information on regulated digital health tools	fda.gov/medical-devices/digital-health

A.17 Glossary of Key Terms

Adoption: The decision to employ an intervention; the proportion of eligible settings or providers that begin using an intervention.
Balancing Measure: A measure that monitors for unintended consequences of an intervention.
CFIR (Consolidated Framework for Implementation Research): A comprehensive framework for assessing barriers and facilitators to implementation across five domains.
De-implementation: The process of reducing or stopping the use of low-value or harmful practices.
Effectiveness: The impact of an intervention on outcomes in real-world settings.

Efficacy: The impact of an intervention on outcomes under ideal, controlled conditions.
Fidelity: The degree to which an intervention is delivered as intended.
Health Disparities: Negative differences in health linked to social, economic, and environmental disadvantages.
Health Equity: The state in which everyone has a fair and just opportunity to be as healthy as possible.
Health Inequities: Modifiable differences in access to facilities and services associated with social disadvantages.
Implementation: The process of putting an intervention into practice.
Implementation Science: The scientific study of methods to promote the systematic uptake of evidence-based practices into routine care.
Implementation Strategy: A specific method, technique, or activity used to enhance adoption, implementation, and sustainability.
Maintenance: The degree to which an intervention is sustained over time after external support ends.
Outcome Measure: A measure of the ultimate result you are trying to achieve.
PDSA Cycle: Plan-Do-Study-Act; an iterative method for testing and refining changes.
Penetration: The integration of an intervention into routine practice; the proportion of eligible patients receiving the intervention.
Process Measure: A measure of whether the intervention is being delivered as intended.
Quality Improvement (QI): Systematic efforts to improve healthcare processes and outcomes.
RE-AIM: A framework for planning and evaluating implementation across five dimensions: Reach, Effectiveness, Adoption, Implementation, Maintenance.
Reach: The proportion of the target population that participates in or receives an intervention.
Run Chart: A graph that displays data over time to detect patterns and trends.
Scalability: The ability to expand an intervention to reach more people or settings.
SMART Aim: An aim statement that is Specific, Measurable, Achievable, Relevant, and Time-bound.
SQUIRE 2.0: Standards for Quality Improvement Reporting Excellence; guidelines for reporting QI work.
Sustainability: The degree to which an intervention is maintained over time after external support ends.

A.18 Final Checklist: Is Your QI Project Ready?

Before You Start:

☐ Problem is important to patients, residents, and institution
☐ Team is assembled with appropriate stakeholders
☐ Current process is mapped and understood
☐ Root causes are identified
☐ SMART aim statement is written
☐ Measures are defined (outcome, process, balancing)
☐ Baseline data collection plan is in place
☐ Faculty mentor is engaged
☐ Institutional approval obtained (if needed)
☐ Equity considerations incorporated

During Implementation:

☐ PDSA cycles are documented
☐ Data are collected and displayed over time
☐ Team meets regularly to review progress
☐ Barriers are identified and addressed
☐ Stakeholders are kept informed
☐ Adaptations are documented

After Implementation:

☐ Results are analyzed and interpreted
☐ Lessons learned are documented
☐ Sustainability plan is in place
☐ Handoff to permanent owner is complete
☐ Results are presented and/or published
☐ MOC credit is obtained (if applicable)

Epilogue

The Health Sciences Implementation Blueprint

is more than a handbook. It is a practical invitation to see every clinical setting, every workflow, and every patient encounter as an opportunity to close the gap between what is known and what is done.

Its central message is simple but profound: better is possible. Progress in healthcare does not begin with perfection; it begins with disciplined curiosity, clear thinking, and the willingness to improve what already exists.

When clinicians treat data as a catalyst for action, they begin to transform information into insight, insight into design, and design into better care.

This is the promise of embedded design. Improvement is strongest when it is built into the daily fabric of practice, not added as an afterthought. In that spirit, the handbook encourages learners and clinicians to work inside real systems, with real constraints, and with real teams, so that evidence becomes routine, equity becomes intentional, and sustainability becomes expected.

The future of health sciences will belong to those who can combine evidence with execution, systems thinking with compassion, and innovation with accountability. This handbook is written to help you become one of those people—***to notice what is possible, design for what matters, and help make better the norm rather than the exception***

BETTER IS POSSIBLE. AND YOU ARE THE ONE TO MAKE IT HAPPEN.

About the Author

Dr. Kesling is a health care executive, academician, and clinician with over five decades of experience across a broad range of organizations in both the public and private sector working with local, state, and federal agencies. Half of those years were in collaborating, promoting, and nurturing in academic environments serving as a faculty at academic health science centers' Schools of Medicine, Nursing and Health Professions and the Executive Dean of a College of Health Sciences at the Texas Medical Center, Houston.

Contributor, Draft Recommendation for Standard E Code Grouping for Morbidity and Mortality Systems. Contributor for surveillance data sets. National Center on Injury Prevention and Control (NCIPC) of the Centers for Disease Control and Prevention and the Morbidity Classification Branch of the National Center for Health Statistics (NCHS) with the Council of the Injury Control and Emergency Health Services Section of the American Public Health Association. October 1995.

Contributor for the National Highway Safety Administration's EMS White Paper 1996: established program guidelines and recommendations related to the current and future state of emergency medical services

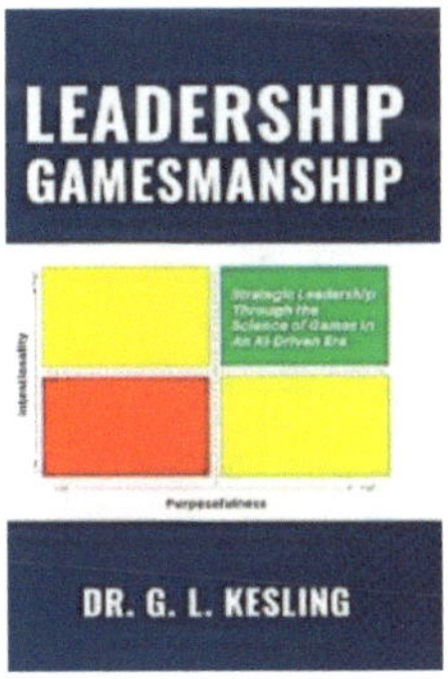

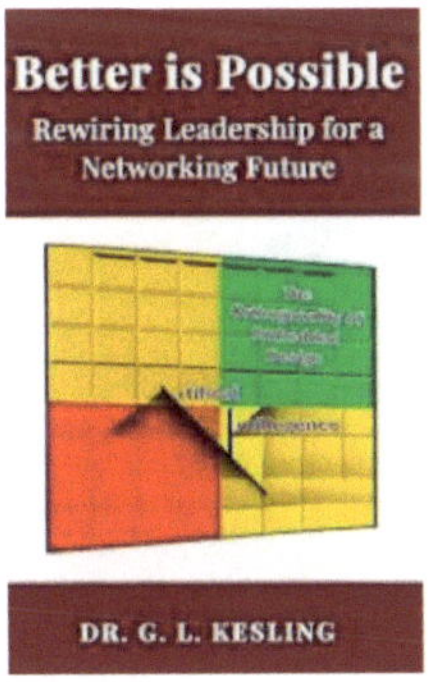

Kesling, G. L. (2025). *Leadership Gamesmanship: Strategic Leadership Through the Science of Games in an AI-Driven Era.* Dr. G. L. Kesling (Publisher). ISBN-13: 979-8900566153. Published September 16, 2025.

Kesling, G. L. (2025). *Better is Possible: Rewiring Leadership for a Networking Future.* Independently published. ISBN-13: 979-8264813726. Published September 10, 2025.

www.ingramcontent.com/pod-product-compliance
Lightning Source LLC
LaVergne TN
LVHW051154210926
848486LV00005B/276